MAGGIE DOWNIE

Take Steps to
Relieve Pain
& Improve
Your Life

Enjoy Moving !

Maggie D.

KEEP
MOVING

D1379717

Enjoy Mary!

Megan

Publishing Services provided by Paper Raven Books

Printed in the United States of America

First Printing, 2018

Paperback ISBN= 978-1-7326075-0-7
Hardback ISBN= 978-1-7326075-1-4

Dedication:

My Two Grandmas

Ruth Sparano Hale & Lillian Fouhey Downie

TABLE OF CONTENTS

Introduction   1

    My Pain Story   3

    Pilates and the Movement Method   6

    What I Learned from My Grandparents   9

Section One: How Pain Works   13

    Chapter 1: Understanding Pain   15

    Chapter 2: Fitness Misconceptions That
Hold You Back   41

    Chapter 3: You Are Not Alone in This   59

Section Two: This Is Your Body, and You Only
Get One!   69

    Chapter 4: How Your Body Works   75

    Chapter 5: How Your Body Parts Integrate
and Work Together   97

    Chapter 6: Laying the Groundwork   129

    Chapter 7: Common Exercise Concerns   157

Section Three: The Moves   171

    Chapter 8: Happy Feet   175

    Chapter 9: Happy Hips & Low Back   191

    Chapter 10: Happy Neck & Shoulders   219

Resources   245

Acknowledgements   247

Works Cited   249

Thank you for choosing *Keep Moving*. It is the culmination of years of research and experience working with clients, both injured and non-injured. My PEEPs in Motion partner, Cate Vallone and I found that many of our clients were living with similar types of pain. That inspired us to create Workshops for Wellness, designed to educate people about common pain and the movements that can help unravel discomfort. In time, those workshops led to the idea for this book and became the backbone of the exercises provided. At the back of the book, you will find links to more resources. I truly hope the information helps you feel better in your own body and provides a sense of control over what happens to your body. You do have control.

Ethan Harper is a freelance illustrator and animator currently residing in the super fancy city of Los Angeles, California. He met the author while attending high school together in their home state of Connecticut—staying good friends with her ever since—and was excited for and remains humbled by the opportunity given him to help bring this book to life. He also looks forward to attempting to apply Maggie's excellent advice to his own daily routine, especially after discovering over the course of their collaboration exactly how desperately he needs to.

More examples of Ethan's art—and occasional further ramblings—can be found on various social media outlets (Instagram and Twitter, primarily) under @ethancharper.

INTRODUCTION

If you're reading this, you want a life without chronic pain. Perhaps you've lived with it for so long that a pain-free life seems like a pipe dream, but it is possible to feel good in your body. I know how frustrating, exhausting, and aggravating constant discomfort can be, but know that pain is not guaranteed to be permanent. My own experiences with pain, my clients' journeys, and a great deal of research make me confident that you can alleviate the pain that permeates your life if you keep moving.

I'm trained in the Pilates Method and have been teaching since 2005. I became a Pilates instructor by accident, although looking back I should have considered a career in health and fitness when picking colleges. Movement has always been a part of my life. As a child, I enjoyed dance and sports. In college when doing theater, I encouraged fellow actors to exercise during rehearsal breaks on the basis "your body is your tool." (Fortunately, they didn't kick me out of drama club.) Eventually, my full-time desk job at a museum disrupted my regular workout routine. Having put on a little weight and missing movement, I bought a membership to a local gym. They offered a Pilates class, so every week on Wednesday nights you would find me there. A year later when the instructor left, the gym asked if I would get certified and take over the class. Thus began a change in career and a future I hadn't anticipated but love. Pilates provides the movement that has always fulfilled me and gives me tools to help others.

Though one of my specialties is injured populations, I see a broad range of clients. They all have one thing in common: everyone, no matter how fit or how old, experiences pain. Maybe they showed up at my door with sciatica or chronic back pain, or after reaching for something they aggravated their shoulder, or they suffer from rheumatoid arthritis that has been progressing over time, or they tore a tendon while running. They show up to move because moving makes them feel better. As a lover of Pilates, I think the Pilates method is a wonderful way to move that can enhance any movement you love. I also know it isn't the only option. In general, I'm fascinated by movement and enjoy the creativity that comes with helping people find ways to reduce pain. I've been in pain myself and had to find my way out of it with a team of helpers, including Pilates instructors, chiropractors, sports medicine doctors, physical therapists, massage therapists, and acupuncturists. We live in a world with a number of tools at our fingertips that can help us recover from pain; the difficult part is finding which tools work for *you*.

When something hurts, movement is where I turn to first, but it doesn't come to mind for everyone. A close relative who is nearing 80 has lived with Charcot-Marie-Tooth—a neurological disorder resulting in weakness in the legs, foot deformities, and eventual muscle atrophy in the hands that affect fine motor skills. As he noticed his fine motor skills declining and pain in his hands increasing, he went for medical advice and was told he could have a surgery to help. He wasn't interested in surgery or the recovery that comes with it. I suggested he try two or three very simple hand exercises and stretches. He began doing them daily and within weeks felt his motor skills improve and his pain diminish. This story is not meant to suggest that I know more than a doctor, but it reflects that movement is an option to try before undergoing surgery, yet no one suggested this method, which has minimal recovery time and almost no risk of infection.

Right now, you may not love moving and may feel intimidated by the idea of movement. You may be scared to move. You may have never been a regular mover, so that option doesn't come naturally to you. Let's change that together. Change may take time, and it probably won't be easy, but with the right guide, mindset, and tools, you can take back your life and minimize the need for pills and surgeries to conquer chronic pain. Understanding how pain works and what is happening in your body is the key to unraveling pain. Pain, for all the frustrations it causes, can be a motivator, after all. It's time to learn how it can be a tool, not a hindrance.

My Pain Story

A few years ago, I eagerly joined four female friends and their children at the opening of a trampoline park. It was meant to be a fun break and a chance to feel like a kid again. Who doesn't want to jump around with childlike giddiness for an afternoon? My friends bounced once or twice and cautiously dismounted. They had both the wisdom and the diminished bladder control that often accompanies motherhood signaling them to retreat. Not blessed with children or wisdom, I persisted.

Jumping in the air, I was suddenly 10 years old again. The distance between me and the trampoline increased on every bounce as did

3

my exhilaration; hyped-up on endorphins, each jump increased my confidence. I was physically as old as when I'd walked into the park, but I felt scads younger. Normally, my body feels heavy and dense, but with these magical springs beneath me, movement felt effortless and buoyant as if I could float, flip, and fly forever. All notions of my personal safety dissolved. However, my real age was growing more apparent as I ignored a mild twinge in my back, surprisingly sore quads, a buckle in my knees, and a stiffening neck.

On what became my final forward flip, I did not fully rotate. My butt landed where my feet should have, and I fell backwards, causing my chin to slam into my chest. The subsequent bounce snapped my head back like a frantic Pez dispenser. It happened so fast that there was no time to brace or protect my body. Instead of being rewarded with a tasty candy, I bit my tongue. Everything hurt. It was too late to heed all the warning signs my body had given me. The springs I'd loved only a moment ago now felt like torture. All I wanted was stillness, but I was stuck to these undulating buoys. Fear filled my thoughts as I tried to determine how severe or permanent the damage was. Had I just snapped my neck? Could I wiggle my fingers? Could I feel my legs?

As the last adult on the trampoline, supine and still, tortured by the bounding of gleeful children effortlessly bouncing as they hopped past my limp body, I recognized the need to complete the monumental task of crawling two feet to the edge of this acrobatic hell. The pain was intense. I was embarrassed. I told no one, attempting to play it cool. Admitting I'm in pain is never easy for me. If only I could freeze time and suspend the motion of everyone and everything while I made my next move. Splayed out and clearly suffering from whiplash, I had to make a decision about what to do next while working around this new agony in a world that continued revolving. Realizing that all my parts could move brought a bit of relief, but I was about to embark on months of movement therapy to help heal my upper back and neck. Fortunately, as a Pilates instructor, I had many of the tools I would need at my fingertips.

This is not a book of panaceas, and it is certainly not going to solve all your problems. Claiming I have that power would be misleading. This book contains suggestions on how to control and reduce chronic pain based on current research and my knowledge and experience as a Pilates instructor. I use anecdotes from my personal experiences with pain and movement, and I share over a decade's worth of learning from my clients' experiences. You may always have some level of pain, but you also have options for managing those sensations. It is possible to move forward without pain or at the very least with less pain.

The goal of this book it to provide tips, recommendations, and options to help anyone reduce, get out of, and stay out of pain. Movement is scientifically proven to diminish pain, depression, and the general malaise my Italian grandmother calls *moosha moosh*. Moving should be our ideal way to prevent pain, but that is frequently not the case. Sometimes a pill seems easier when we need a quick fix. Sometimes movement hurts, and we are afraid. Sometimes we simply do not know where to begin. It is time to change that perspective and to gain the tools and confidence that will enable you to choose movement no matter what is happening in your body. You should always talk to your doctor before starting a new exercise or movement routine, but if your doctor suggests you stop moving entirely, get a second opinion. The research is fairly definitive that inactivity makes our mindset and our injuries worse.

You know your body better than anyone. You know it better than I do. You know it better than your doctor, your mom, and your greatest love. They understand what the world, movement, and pain feel like in their own bodies; only you truly understand yours. Sometimes in our hectic lives we lose touch with our body, like a long-lost friend. Reconnecting will help you feel better when you figure out what exactly your body needs.

Pilates and the Movement Method

Before physical therapists formed a professional association in 1921, Joe Pilates was developing and teaching functional, rehabilitative movement to injured soldiers in WWI. Later, he employed his methods to rehabilitate and strengthen dancers in New York City. While I'm an advocate for all types of movement, I'll mention Pilates frequently since that is the style of movement I'm the most familiar with. While I'm not a physical therapist, the Pilates approach I'm trained in is geared toward safety, injury prevention, and rehabilitation. I have studied the body extensively, always hunting for answers when what would be expected to work doesn't get the job done.

Pilates often looks for subtle positional changes we can make in the body to feel more comfortable or to find a way to move that doesn't cause discomfort. Pilates attempts to create a strong, stable, balanced core with long limber limbs, neutral joints, and the ability to breathe deeply and free of restriction. It seeks balance in the body so that every part is working in unison to stabilize us as we sit, stand, or walk around, searching for quality over quantity in movement. Pilates has big moves and subtle adjustments to enhance the big moves. Whenever I have been injured, it has been my ability to engage in micro-movements (very small, subtle moves in the body) without feeling like I'm not doing "enough" that has helped the most.

Pilates has enabled me to build deep, core strength that gives me confidence to move safely. The method has made me more in tune with my body and all the movements I love doing. While it would be great if we could all start from this place, it's never too late to learn. Pilates is also not the only answer; the concepts presented in this book come from a variety of movement styles. Joe Pilates borrowed from yoga, gymnastics, and even animal behavior. It's exploratory, as any movement that is going to help you reduce pain needs to be. Any type of movement can help heal. Yoga or tai chi can teach you to be more in tune with your body. The Feldenkrais Method emphasizes micro-movements. Running can help burn off steam. When we are in pain, we need to move. Like anything in life, we'll be more likely to continue moving if we enjoy it, so find a modality that brings you pleasure. We don't need an expensive gym or a Pilates class to experience relief.

We often ignore our bodies and have a plethora of good excuses: deadlines, kids, stress, time. Life gets in the way of making the best health choices. The problem with pushing through pain or skipping movement is that the body has certain basic needs in order to function. When those needs are not met, its automatic response is to behave like a jilted friend. Most likely, it started by delivering subtle or perhaps even passive-aggressive hints, but we brushed them aside to prioritize everything else that seemed more pressing at the time. Once in chronic pain, the body, like our forgotten friend, requires some quality attention.

Build a relationship with your body. Be attentive. You are likely willing to work on relationships with your spouse, your parents, your children, your friends, but in that mix, you often put yourself last. Perhaps you're not even on the list. You have one body. It has the potential to take you anywhere you want to go and to enable you to reach every goal you set, but you have to support and pay attention to your body just as you would support and pay attention to anyone who is important in your life.

That's why becoming aware of the feedback our body provides throughout the day is beneficial. Unless we experience an acute, sudden injury, we probably had a twinge of pain before it developed into something worse. When we don't listen to the signals long enough, one of two things happen: The signals either shut down, feeling ignored, which means we could be damaging something without realizing it, because we continue to follow a pattern that is actually harmful. Or they get louder, intensifying the pain sensation. Both events eventually lead to increased pain. When we listen to our bodies, the systems inside start operating better together, like a highly functional family. When we work with our bodies rather than against it, we are rewarded with ease of movement and agility.

Think back to a time you hurt your little finger, stubbed your toe, or bit your tongue. How much did that affect your daily life every time you used that part of your body? We tend to take our body parts for granted until we are in pain, then we notice them with every move. A small part of us can become a major nuisance. That pain influences the choices we make, including how we sit, walk, and talk, and ultimately alters our daily lives. Pain can make it difficult to move, but we can make adjustments to ease our discomfort. We all need to be less sedentary, since the frequency with which we sit is often part of our pain cycle. As the title of this book indicates, my goal is to have you *keep moving*. This is why I've included small movement breaks throughout the book. When you come across one, take a moment to read through it and then get up and give it a try. They are added to help you experience and understand a particular concept in your own body. Remember, the key is to move, so don't worry about perfecting each exercise.

The chapters that follow are meant to provide a basic understanding of how your body works and to offer multiple, practical exercises that can help you feel better. A particular exercise may work for 90 percent of people, yet it may not be the one that works for you. That's okay. Trust yourself. One of the most important goals of this book is to help you trust your decisions about your movement more than you do now.

What I Learned from My Grandparents

My grandparents exchanged love letters between Connecticut and the South Pacific during WWII. The notes were signed "Somewhere at Sea" by my grandfather and smacked with a pink lipstick kiss from my grandmother. He'd dream about future Christmases at home with her, going out with friends, traveling together, and raising their future children. A typical day at home—imagined by my grandfather while cruising the hot, humid seas of the South Pacific—included mowing the grass, cooking together, going dancing, playing Frisbee at Devil's Hopyard, winning at bowling so the other couple would have to buy drinks, and the longings of nearly every youthful newlywed.

By the time I was born, my grandma with the full, pink lips had been wheelchair-bound and bedridden for 30 years. In her 30s, she was diagnosed with rheumatoid arthritis. The disease crept up on her, but the change from mobility to immobility was sudden. She maintained an incredible attitude, and she never seemed to let it get her down, though I'm sure she had her moments. Today, she would have had a healthier life, since they have better medication for rheumatoid arthritis. She died when I was four from complications with a medication. My grandfather never said anything bad about my grandma to me, but he would sometimes tell me that what bothered him most was knowing that if she had exercised more, she might have had more mobility. The doctor had told her if she moved as much as possible, she may not need a wheelchair and could possibly walk with braces. She needed to exercise, and she chose not to because it hurt too much. My grandpa wished she would have worked through some of that pain, so they could have had a higher quality of life together.

I can't judge her. I never felt her pain. I don't have arthritis, and I can't imagine how she hurt, but I know movement is a simple way to improve everything in life, including emotional and physical pain. Without moving, my grandma descended even faster into a life of constant discomfort with hands crippled into crumpled-up balls. My grandfather's words stuck with me. I believe that if she had moved, she could have altered her own fate. Since rheumatoid arthritis is genetic, I worried throughout my childhood that I might get it and become bedridden. Today, I wouldn't wind up in bed, but I still worry. I move as a precaution to safeguard my future. I want my body to be as mobile as possible for as long as possible. I want the active life my grandparents dreamed about in the letters they shared during wartime.

My other grandma also faced a serious health challenge early in her life when she contracted polio at age nine. In the hospital, she was strapped to a wooden board and immobilized in bed for six months. The nurses regularly wheeled dead bodies destroyed by polio past her bed. When she was released from the hospital, she was weak from atrophy and immobilization and was left with one leg shorter than the other. The doctors told her mother that she would never walk again. Her mother wouldn't accept that outcome. She had six children, and her immigrant mentality was fixated on a better life for her child. She forced my grandma to start moving right away even though it hurt. She massaged her legs day and night. The internet could not confirm she was doing the right thing, but there was nothing to lose. When I was a kid and my grandma was in her 60s, she walked three miles a day, even in the rain. She clung to movement and to this day swears by it for keeping her healthy. She is 92 now. She doesn't walk three miles anymore. She gets tuckered easily (did you notice I said she is over 90?), although her doctor recently told her walking will keep her energy up. I've seen her get up and down from the floor with ease to grab me a cookbook on the bottom shelf, and she has sat on my large stability ball comfortably and laughed. On her 89th birthday, she even wiggled in and out of an igloo.

There are lots of reasons I move. I feel better physically, mentally, and emotionally, and I find physical activity fun. I want freedom, and movement provides that. Most of all, though, I want to be like my grandma when I'm 92: vivacious, active, and still moving. She is my inspiration. Her story motivates me to move. The different lives of my grandmothers inspire me in different ways, but I want to be the one who is 90 and still moving. I believe we always have a choice, and I choose to move. You can, too.

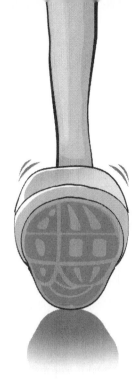

SECTION ONE:
HOW PAIN WORKS

CHAPTER 1: UNDERSTANDING PAIN

"If you can't fly, then run. If you can't run, then walk. If you can't walk, then crawl. But whatever you do, you have to keep moving forward."

—Martin Luther King Jr.

Bombarded by headlines about depression, celebrity deaths, and the opioid health crisis, our society is being tormented by chronic pain. America is in the throes of a public health emergency. Five million deaths worldwide are linked to inactivity, which increases the risk of non-communicable diseases including coronary heart disease, type 2 diabetes, and breast and colon cancers.[1] Opioid overdose kills over 33,000 people per year in

---

1 Lee, I-Min et al., "Effect of Physical Inactivity on Major Non-Communicable Diseases Worldwide: An Analysis of Burden of Disease and Life Expectancy," The Lancet 380, no. 9838 (July 2012): 219–29, https://doi.org/10.1016/S0140-6736(12)61031-9.

the United States. Often, those drugs were sought or introduced to combat chronic pain. Even if we stop prescribing opioids, the problem persists because people remain in pain.

If you are one of the one-in-three Americans living with chronic pain, *Keep Moving* is designed for you. Whether you are faced with a sudden, acute injury from a car accident or sport, have developed pain over time from sitting at a desk or engaging in repetitive motions, have started to feel the effects of life's general wear and tear on the body, or suffer from a disease like fibromyalgia, rheumatoid arthritis, or neuropathy from cancer treatments, the one thing we know for sure is that *movement will help*.

You will never have a life without pain. That is impossible, and you wouldn't want it. Pain is protective. It is intended to be a guide and serves a purpose. Pain keeps us alive and prevents serious injury by warning us to stop drinking a cup of scalding tea or reminding us to put on the oven mitt when we reach for the hot pan. Normally, we consider pain a negative. The ouch-factor hurts and that seems bad. But pain is a brilliant mechanism for our survival. When functioning properly, pain tells us to remove ourselves from an unsafe situation. Pain is a part of life, but should not be a permanent state of being. The goal of this book is to help ensure you are not trapped in chronic, debilitating, life-altering pain.

In order to minimize chronic pain, we need four skills.

1) **Understanding.** Having a basic concept of how pain works can help us recognize what we need to reduce pain. A basic understanding of our own anatomy is a key factor in feeling better, because we get more out of movement when we understand why it is helpful. Ask questions throughout the process. You will have a better chance of

improving if you have confidence in your practitioners and if you understand why and how what you are doing can help.

2) **Listening.** We must learn to listen to the body, both when it is signaling that we are in pain and when an action feels good. Learning to recognize what hurts, what heals, and what provides relief is essential. Part of listening involves trusting what we feel. If you have ever been to therapy to heal a broken personal relationship, you know listening to your partner is key to a successful relationship. It's the same thing with our bodies; we need to listen to them to have a successful mind/body partnership.

3) **Responding.** Based on the feedback from our bodies, we need to alter movements and patterns that cause pain. We can make a conscious effort to adjust our posture and position in daily life, seeking more variety in movement. Our bodies were designed to move, but when our movements are repetitive and lack variation, we develop strain. We can make changes throughout our day that improve our lives and reduce pain in the body.

4) **Moving.** Immobility breeds discomfort and spreads pain. We have to find ways to move more. Some of these can be lifestyle changes that make it easier to fit movement into our daily life. While we need to find time to exercise, we must also ensure that we are selecting quality, functional moves that are best for our body so that we utilize the limited time we have wisely.

To gain these skills, we must question everything we think we know about movement and the body, particularly old paradigms like "No pain, no gain." Having a basic understanding of how our body works encourages us to make better choices for our personal needs. Be comfortable challenging convention and asking anyone providing treatment why they have selected a particular route of treatment for us.

A 2015 study led by Marie Hoeger Bement, PT, PhD, and Kathleen Sluka, PT, PhD, found that after surveying accredited physical therapy (PT) programs only 63 percent of schools self-reported that they felt they adequately educated students on pain topics. In the same survey, only 6 percent (11 of the 167 schools that participated), reported having a dedicated class on pain or pain theory.[2] At first, this might seem obvious. After all, isn't everything physical therapists learn about related to pain and how to get people out of pain? While pain is certainly a regular topic in physical therapy programming, this same survey found only an average of 31 hours were spent on pain in coursework with total hours ranging from 5 to 115 depending on the school's program. Even some of the top-rated physical therapy programs in the United States do not offer a dedicated course on pain. That is the equivalent of a teacher never taking a course on learning theory or an electrician never learning about electrical theory—both dedicated courses individuals entering those fields are required to take early in their training.

Luckily, this is starting to change. Seth Hagymasi, PT, DPT, OCS explains that the majority of research on pain, pain science, and pain therapeutic neuroscience has been conducted in the last 10 to 15 years.[3] Hegymasi doesn't aggressively push clients through pain. He tries to educate patients about moving back slowly into motions that once hurt sometimes using an analogy of a soda bottle. Once a soda bottle has been shaken (like

---

2 American Physical Therapy Association, "Many PT Programs Describe Their Pain Management Education as Not 'Adequate'," PT in Motion, March 3, 2015, www.apta.org/PTinMotion/News/2015/3/3/PTPainEducation/.

3 Supervisor of Spine Rehabilitation at UCONN Health Center in Farmington, Connecticut and adjunct faculty of Physical Therapy at the University of Hartford.

our nervous system in pain), if you open the soda quickly, it explodes, makes a mess, and is undrinkable. If you open it slowly, the soda is different. It might be a little flat, but you can drink it. After experiencing chronic pain, even after proper treatment and therapy, we are going to be different, perhaps slightly less carbonated, but that is okay if we can still do everything we want and need to do. Ideally, through the process, we are more aware of our pain threshold, better understand what types of movement cause us pain, and have tools to alter posture and behavior so that we are less likely to return to a state of chronic pain.

In the words of professor and physical therapist Beth Fisher, "Physical therapy in general is not a one-size-fits-all approach, whether orthopedic or neurological. There are too many variables that make individuals different—psychological issues, pain tolerance, how important it is for them to get back. Intervention really needs to be tailored to that person because there is just so much to apply one approach to each person."[4] She also points out that we all need to realize what motivates us. Practitioners need to find the motivator to best help heal patients, but as patients we have to figure out what it is we really want. Maybe we want to be out of pain. Perhaps our goal is to get back to running or get up and down off the floor. Maybe you can live with the pain you are in, but the limp you have developed embarrasses you and you want the limp to go away. Figuring out what your individual, real goal or motivator is will help you stick to a program. And sticking with a program will help you reach the goal. Then you need to explore what types of movements yield the best results for you.

---

4 PhD, PT, FAPTA, a Professor of Clinical Physical Therapy in the Division of Biokinesiology and Physical Therapy at the University of Southern California and Director of the Neuroplasticity & Imaging Laboratory.

I wish I could promise that if you do everything this book suggests that your current pain will go away forever. No one can promise that. Nothing is a guarantee. What I do know is that if you incorporate the suggestions that work for you from this book, you will gain some control over your pain without doing anything invasive. Noticing pain signals earlier will help to prevent pain before it begins or to reduce the severity when it occurs. Finding positions that provide relief will give you a much-needed sense of ease. You will gain a better understanding of your body and what it needs to function optimally.

Simple strategies are key and available. Pain will pop up at different times in our lives. Dealing with the discomfort is still a nuisance, but in knowing how to "fix" the problem, we regain control of the body that was for a while under the dominion of chronic pain. Pain is never any fun and is made worse when we feel trapped. Pain strikes stillness and stiffness within us. Once you learn the tools that empower you, pain becomes an inconvenience, not debilitating. You absolutely do not have to fight pain with pain. If you learn anything from this book, please absorb that. Unraveling pain does not have to be miserable. Movement does not need to be agonizing. You are not alone on your journey with pain.

If you Google "neck," "shoulder," or "knee," the Google gods presume the next word you will type is "pain." We are a world searching for answers to chronic discomfort. *Keep Moving* will lay out common myths and misconceptions about exercise. Reconsidering long-assumed ideas about pain and movement will provide a world of possibility. After a stimulating, educational race through the anatomy that will help you understand what your body needs in order for you to live with less pain, we will lay the foundation for exercises that can strengthen you and build stamina to withstand the unexpected challenges of life.

Movement provides so many daily pleasures. Breathing is movement. Chewing, swallowing, digesting is movement. It gets you through your day and enables all your interactions with the world around you. You must keep moving for lifelong independence. The more mobile you stay throughout life, the more choices you have. This book is designed to provide a new understanding of your body, a different way to think about and incorporate movement, and a guide for you to live with less pain. If you are not experiencing pain, the goal is to maintain the status quo and prevent future aches. If you are experiencing chronic pain, the goal is to give you the tools to diminish discomfort as much as possible. The information in this book is based on the most up-to-date scientific studies available. But the science of human movement, anatomy, and injuries is rapidly changing and growing. We are always learning more.

If you want to feel better but aren't sure where to begin, this book can help you chart your first steps in your path toward wellness. Along the way, I hope you laugh and learn. Relieving discomfort and living pain-free is an ever-changing process. Let's try to enjoy the process together.

Which Type of Pain is Bringing You Down?

Pain can strike us at any point. It can be sudden or creep into our body over time. At different ages and places in our lives, we may experience different types of pain. Children are endlessly knocking into objects and actually building up their nervous system, learning to sense themselves in space. A small but growing number of teens and young adults experience Amplified Musculoskeletal Pain Syndrome, a nervous system disorder that causes incapacitating pain with no sign of tissue damage. Four times more prevalent in young girls than boys, it is believed that the increased prevalence may be due to over scheduling, stress, and type A personalities.[5] Other teens and young adults experience injuries through sports. By middle age, we may start to notice aches and pains we never had before. Maybe we are stiff getting out of bed, and the activities we used to enjoy take more out of us and require longer recovery periods. All the bumps and bruises we have accumulated through life seem to nag us by the time we hit 60. Seniors ages 65 and up are more active than ever, which is why they are motivated to eliminate the pain getting in their way. If we have arthritis or another inflammatory illness, the pain may become more debilitating with age.

Beyond the typical life trajectory, we also have to deal with injuries throughout life. When it comes to healing an injury, we often want the quick fix. A pill that masks the pain seems especially tempting. Don't get me wrong; pills can be useful and helpful, and we are lucky to live in a time where medicine is an option. However, the problem is never that simple or that easy and neither is the solution. Fortunately, we have tools within our own body to help us heal, manage, and (ideally) eliminate pain. Understanding the difference between types of pain matters, because the way we wound up in pain in the first place plays a role in the way we will resolve the discomfort.

Most likely, you are experiencing acute or chronic pain. Acute pain is the result of a sudden injury, such as twisting your ankle stepping off the sidewalk or getting whiplash from a car accident. Surgery may be required, but limited rest followed by movement and physical therapy with proper guidance and exercise choices should resolve acute pain. (Although that doesn't mean the fear of its return disappears.)

---

5 Sarah Vander Schaaff, "The Strange Pain that Can Overcome Kids, Especially High-Achieving Teenage Girls," *The Washington Post*, August 6, 2017.

Chronic pain, on the other hand, lingers. The pain doesn't seem to go away and has lasted over three months. We can feel like we are chasing the pain, and seeing doctors or various healers with no definitive answer. Determining the cause can be a challenge; maybe it started with an acute injury or maybe there is no clear explanation for how it started. If you have been experiencing pain in your body for more than three months, you should seek medical attention. Hopefully, you already have, but if nothing seems to be improving, it's time to go back for answers. Chronic pain may develop for a variety of unknown reasons but usually stems from one of three main culprits:

An Unhealed Acute Injury

The neck still nags you since the accident. The ankle never felt right after it twisted, and now your knee hurts all the time. Ideally, the right exercises, massage, and other modalities should help reduce or eliminate this pain. And the faster you work toward a resolution, the better.

Repetitive Strain, General Wear and Tear, or Faulty Movement Patterns

We all face this issue if we live long enough. Maybe we never totally fixed an acute injury and we ended up with a limp that worsened over time. Perhaps we always put more pressure on one leg or hip and now we have arthritis that is worse on one side. Maybe from years of repeatedly lifting heavy objects, we developed spinal stenosis. When the cause originated from a faulty pattern, it can be undone by learning new patterns. As with most pain, the earlier you attend to a bad pattern, the better. "Faulty," "bad," or "wrong" for terms about movement bother me. On some level if you are moving it shouldn't be wrong. If that movement is causing pain, however, something needs to be adjusted. Movement itself is not right or wrong. We can have better or worse form. But we really need to ask, "Does it hurt or feel good?" We alter our movements from "wrong" to "right" in order to get out of pain, to prevent a repetitive action that is likely to lead to pain, or to encourage particular muscles to fire and help a person feel the movement in a different way.

Autoimmune or Other Diseases

Sometimes there was never an injury or a faulty pattern. Rheumatoid arthritis, neuropathy that developed from cancer treatment or diabetes, Lyme disease, or a host of other illnesses developed into the pain you feel now. This can be trickier, because the movement we once loved may feel like it depletes us instead of providing energy. But movement doesn't have to be eliminated. We need to explore and listen to the body. One helpful strategy includes micro-movements, which we'll learn more about later.

The Pain Loop

Scientists don't completely understand the nervous system yet, especially when it comes to chronic pain. Our brains have the ability to trap us in a pain loop, telling us we are in pain, even if we have no clear physical reason to be in pain. Please do not take this to mean that your pain is all in your head. Whether you should or should not be in pain according to a test or imaging results is of minimal consequence. If your brain thinks you are in pain, you are going to be in pain. If your brain believes a particular situation is your reality, it is your reality. Luckily, brains can learn new tricks.

In 2006, cognitive neuroscientist Henrik Ehrsson and a team of researchers developed the Rubber Hand Experiment, which revealed how our brains comprehend body ownership, the ability to differentiate the parts of the body that are ours from the parts that belong to the rest of the world.[6] Body ownership is how I know the difference between my hand and yours when we hold hands, or how I know my shoes aren't part of my body when I put them on my feet. The Rubber Hand Experiment showed the world that our brains sometimes get confused about what parts belong to us.

In the experiment, a person puts one hand on a table and a rubber hand where their other hand would rest on the table. The actual hand is under the table beneath the rubber hand. Then the experiment administrator uses a feather and simultaneously tickles the rubber hand and the real hand beneath the table for at least 11 seconds. After which the administrator takes a hammer and smashes the rubber hand. Even though the actual hand is safely beneath the table, participants instinctually pull their hand away to save it from the impact it will never receive.

Subjects in the experiment reacted as if the fake rubber hand were their own. They could intellectually tell the hand did not belong to them, but within 11 seconds of feather tickling, they felt as if it were part of their own body. The feeling was so powerful that if harm was going to come to the rubber hand, the participant would pull their own hand away. You are in pain if you think you are in pain, but it is possible, especially if testing shows nothing is wrong with your hip, back, or neck, that your brain crossed some signals. The nervous system can get caught in a pain cycle, becoming more efficient at telling us we are in pain, even if it is erroneous information. Our brains can get stuck on repeat, thinking we are in pain even when our body is healed.

We protect ourselves at all costs. This means that we can do something repeatedly without injury, but once we get hurt during

---

6 New Scientist, "Body Illusions: Rubber Hand Illusion," March 18, 2009, https://www.newscientist.com/article/dn16809-body-illusions-rubber-hand-illusion/.

that task, we become increasingly cautious about that movement. This limits our own mobility going forward. Originally, the pain is good; it's a signal to be gentle and cautious with an injured or inflamed area. But sometimes the signal and nervous system can get too efficient at relaying the pain signal, lowering the threshold for the amount of sensation needed to signal pain and creating faster pathways that relay the pain back and forth between the brain and the body.

Adriaan Louw explains that when we step on a rusty nail, our nervous system spikes our pain sensation to enable us to react and get to safety.[7] After removing the nail from the foot, it may still throb and hurt to remind us the area is healing and we need to be sensitive with it. The pain loop happens when the nervous systems continues to react even after that nail is gone and the wound is healed, signaling pain even though we no longer have any sign of injury. Our body appears fine, but our nervous system is making us feel we have pain. When we get stuck in a loop of fear or when the brain gets confused, it is time to retrain the brain so it knows whose hand is whose, that the nail is gone and we are fully healed, and whether or not it should still be sending out a pain signal. We need to give the brain a new story to tell our body.

The solution to ending the pain loop is simple: start moving. The brain has to relearn that movement does not really hurt. The how and to what degree can require a little more effort and fine tuning, all based on your pain. It is a balance. You and your body are on a team working together. While you are in control, realistically you cannot force your body into a place it is not ready to go. I would likely get injured if I tried to perform *Swan Lake* today.

---

7 Co-founder of the International Spine and Pain Institute, a member of the adjunct faculty at St. Ambrose University, South College, and the University of Nevada Las Vegas.

To unwind pain, we don't simply need movement for the sake of movement (although I don't want to turn you off of that concept), but we may need to analyze our movement. We may require new strategies that minimize stress on our body and joints. If you have developed pain because you are tight somewhere in the body and that tightness interferes with how you move, you need to relearn how you are moving to help redistribute the demands on the joints encouraging the body to work as a team player. Each day is a new day with new opportunity for the brain to learn. What worked for you for a week may need to change. The key is to find what feels good and provides you relief on any given day while also being open to new movement strategies.

The Hope That Heals

Pain can be discouraging, but if one movement does not work for you, another will. It takes time to discover your body's specific needs. With patience, perseverance, and hope, you can form new habits in movement to counteract pain. When someone tells you, "you can't," you will prove them wrong.

When we have a sense of control over what is happening in our bodies, we feel better about the situation. With chronic pain, we almost always have more control than we realize. We often allow pain to control us due to fear, discomfort, lack of time, or convincing ourselves that it is not that bad and we should buck up. I have fallen into this trap myself. I get it. I'm not writing this from a lack of experience. I know that I've never been in your body and that I don't understand your specific pain, but I have lived through my own battle with pain. As someone who has both received and provided care, I know you have likely received unhelpful or potentially harmful advice from someone trying to help.

Physical therapist Beth Fisher found herself in need of therapy for arthritis in her shoulder, which was aggravated by the boxing classes she loved. Her physical therapist's final advice was: "Well, you have to stop boxing." She thought that was a terrible option. "Sure, that is one approach," she said when I spoke with her. Boxing was aggravating her problem, so if she stopped the activity that added stress to the joint, she would feel better. "But when you have an older client invested and committed to exercising, you don't want to mess that up. That is one of the things we are trying to get people to do: commit from a sedentary lifestyle to an active one," she said. So while the advice may have been her cure, it wasn't helpful for her. She didn't want to give up her lifestyle.

My father had a similarly disappointing encounter with his provider. After suffering from an acute knee injury that crept into his hip and back (as pain will do), he was sent to physical therapy. In the course of starting his program, his orthopedic surgeon told him that he didn't need back surgery even though he has degenerative disc disease (DDD) and arthritis. Physical therapy had helped him get out of pain a year before and the surgeon felt it would again. Afterwards, my father saw a well-respected physical therapist in the area who he had seen before and loved. She told him she was certain he needed a spinal fusion and that physical therapy would not help. My father was so deflated. Back at the orthopedic surgeon's office, the doctor told my dad how infrequently spinal fusions help for DDD. In 2009, a study reviewing the clinical trials of back surgery for DDD found that results were modest in pain relief and improved function.[8] The study stated that "the benefits of surgery must be regarded as small."

Don't allow anyone to ever give up hope on you or convince you that you cannot improve. If you happen to wind up in the hands

---

8 Nikolai Bogduk and Gunnar Andersson, "Is Spinal Surgery Effective for Back Pain?" *F1000 Medicine Reports* 1, no. 60 (2009), http://doi.org/10.3410/M1-60.

of a practitioner who tells you that you can't get out of pain, find one who will listen and explain their reasoning. Ask friends until you find an individual who will help you reach your goals.

Our Emotions and Our Pain Are Linked

When discussing pain, we cannot ignore emotions. Chronic pain and emotions are intertwined, although it can lead to a chicken-and-egg question. Did the chronic pain change and affect your emotions? Or did emotions create chronic pain? Most likely, it works both ways. I experienced this when my grandfather was dying. He was one of my favorite people, and I admired, looked up to, and idolized him. When I was a child, he and his mom were my daycare providers, and he had always been a regular part of my life. When he first became ill, I started having heart palpations and low back pain. Part of the cause was physical, since I was spending hours in the car each day to visit him in the hospital and spent long periods sitting beside him and with my family. The back pain was exacerbated by stress and exhaustion. I was in my 20s and was not prone to back pain, yet my lower back ached and stiffened, gripping every time I stood after prolonged sitting. After he died, I had a notable, constricting, deep pain in my chest. I felt the emotion of sadness physically in my body.

Thankfully, the symptoms didn't develop into chronic pain, but we are all living a delusion if we deny the connection between emotions and pain. When we are angry, our hearts race and our jaws tense. When we are nervous, we feel butterflies in our stomachs and start to sweat. The body and the mind are intricately tangled. My clients with chronic low back pain are always worse when they are having a stressful week at work. By pointing out the connection between emotions and physical pain, I'm not trying to minimize anyone's pain. Pain is real, whatever the cause. To better understand the origins of pain, it is important to recognize that there is oftentimes more going on than simply the physical attribute of the pain sensation. It can be a part of the solution.

Stress is a complicated beast. In some situations, stress can make us feel no pain, a beautiful coping mechanism for difficult life situations. The effects of pain under stress is not widely studied on humans, since, as a general rule, we all agree it is immoral to intentionally cause pain or stress to humans. Animal and human studies with small samples have shown that chronic stress increases hyperalgesia (increased sensitivity to pain) and reduces morphine sensitivity.

A small study conducted in Germany in 2013 looked at pain response under stress and discovered stress increased reports of pain in women living with fibromyalgia.[9] This was an unexpected finding, since Benjamin Crettaz and his team expected stress to increase the pain threshold. Think of a solider in a war zone who continues to charge even though he's been shot, or the person who can cut off their own arm to free themselves from a pinned rock. It was presumed that healthy individuals might have an increased pain threshold when responding to stress, but it is not the case. Stress can be hard to define, because it's subjective. While it can clearly reduce or increase our pain depending on the situation, multiple studies support the idea that people dealing with chronic pain have more discomfort under stressful situations.

The pain-stress cycle works both ways. Pain can keep us up, create depression, and produce tension, which causes stress. Stress can also keep us awake at night, create tension, and ultimately cause

---

9 Benjamin Crettaz et al., "Stress-Induced Allodynia—Evidence of Increased Pain Sensitivity in Healthy Humans and Patients with Chronic Pain after Experimentally Induced Psychosocial Stress," *PLOS ONE* 8, no. 8 (2013), https://doi.org/10.1371/journal.pone.0069460.

pain. It's a vicious cycle that we need to break. Find your way to de-stress and decide how often you will do that activity. It will help with your pain.

Though stress plays a role in pain and other ailments, I get annoyed (as I'm sure you do too) when people imply or presume whatever I am going through is stress-related. At the same time, I need to keep an open mind about the role stress plays in my pain. Sometimes pain is physical. Sometimes pain is emotional. Sometimes pain is tension and stress. Most often, it is a combination. If stress is a contributing factor to your pain, how much is it contributing? The question matters, because the answer can alter how you decide to resolve the problem. Even if stress isn't causing your pain, it might be increasing it. You are still in pain. There is still a problem. Don't let anyone brush aside what you are experiencing. Women and African Americans, you especially stand strong. In emergency rooms, African Americans are prescribed painkillers 50 percent less often than white people in non-definitive conditions like back pain or abdominal pain, and women presenting with pain tend to be diagnosed differently than men with the same symptoms.[10] In 2008, a study of 230 family doctors revealed that sample cases of men and women who presented with the same symptoms of a heart attack were diagnosed equally. If stress was listed as a potential symptom, however, only 15 percent of the doctors diagnosed a heart attack for the women while 56 percent diagnosed a heart attack for the men.[11]

If you are a woman, be cautious about allowing your doctor to blame stress for your health or pain. Recognize that it could be a factor, but trust that you know your body. If you are being

---

10 Amanda Holpuch, "Black Patients Half as Likely To Receive Pain Medication as White Patients, Study Finds," *The Guardian*, August 10, 2016.

11 Tara Parker-Pope, "Women's Heart Symptoms Often Blamed on Stress," *The New York Times blog*, October 13, 2008, https://well.blogs.nytimes.com/2008/10/13/just-stress-more-often-diagnosed-in-women/.

honest with yourself that stress is not a main contributing factor, do not be marginalized. Fight for your need for an answer. Sadly, research has shown an innate bias in the medical field. Challenging diseases get diagnosed later in women than men. Crohn's disease takes 12 months on average to diagnose for men but 20 months for women. A rare connective tissue disease takes on average four years to diagnose in men and 12 years in women.[12] When women complain of pain and disease, they are being sidelined. You have every right to stand up for your needs and should not feel bad about it.

Recently, I was having a strange sensation in my heart. It wasn't like the palpitations I'd experienced when I lost my grandfather, and it's difficult to describe. I would suddenly feel very light-headed and my heart would start racing. If I mentioned my symptoms to anybody, the first question they would ask was about my stress level. I started to think I might be crazy. Maybe it was all in my head, but the symptoms were nerve-wracking enough that I went to a doctor. An EKG machine spit out a strip of paper informing me everything was fine. That provided relief but made me wonder what the cause might be. Later that day, I received a note from my endocrinologist saying that my thyroid numbers were off and that I was on the verge of hyperthyroidism. At my appointment with her a few days before, I had mentioned that I was worried about my heart. She wasn't concerned at the time. After receiving the tests later, we altered my thyroid medication, which seemed to alleviate the problem. Perhaps the timing of all it was a fluke, and it wasn't related to my thyroid. Doctors cannot be perfect predictors all the time. They won't always get the answer right. Looking back on it, I feel it is safe to say that my symptoms were not in my head. My symptoms were telling me something was wrong, but I was easily convinced I might be going crazy.

---

12 Maya Dusenbury, "'Everybody Was Telling Me There Was Nothing Wrong,'" *BBC*, May 29, 2018.

Clearly, I still need to learn to trust the sensations my body gives me. I'm on this journey with you. I have lived with my body long enough to know if something isn't right. You have lived in your body long enough to know, too. You always need to be your best advocate. You need to be honest with yourself if stress is the culprit, which can sometimes be hard to see in the moment. But if you know it's not the only factor, trust yourself when the world around you can make you feel senseless when there is no obvious or immediate answer. We once blamed ulcers on stress and left a lot of people in agony, which probably made them pretty stressed. In reality, ulcers are caused by bacteria that can be treated with antibiotics. Until we understood that, though, we blamed the person. We still have a lot to learn about pain. Do not allow your doctor or family to blame stress alone.

Allowing Yourself to Fail is Part of Stopping Pain

In movement, as well as in life, we learn more from our struggles and our failures than our successes. Instead of being exasperated by something we cannot do in the moment, we need to figure out the lesson: what is holding us back, what is getting in our way? Failure can either be frustrating or when the real fun begins. Failure can be maddening because often it reveals a weakness. If we can accept that without judgement, we create room for growth. I see clients all the time struggle to do an exercise because of pain or because their body is not ready for that move yet. The inability to do something presents an opportunity to find clues that will often lead to answers to make you stronger going forward. Had you not tried the exercise, you may not have found the imbalance or weakness that is going to lead to improvement. Even if you are never able to achieve a certain goal, the information you have learned about your body along the way gives you tools and a stronger sense of self if you let it. Every lesson learned supersedes failure.

Some of my best stories come from moments of trial and error. When I hiked Mt. Kilimanjaro, I didn't make it to the top. I had to turn back six hours from the summit after hiking for eight days. That felt like a failure. The next week, an Irish woman my age died hiking the same mountain. Hearing that news made me reconsider whether my decision to turn back really counted as a failure. I didn't make it to the top, but I still had a wonderful adventure. I realized that I had achieved a new personal best, hiking over 17,000 feet in altitude, and I learned that everyone else in my life thinks what I did was fantastic. It was only me that ever saw the failure.

Mark Twain wrote, "It is not in the least likely that any life has ever been lived which was not a failure in the secret judgment of the person who lived it." Our failures and successes are in part based on how we perceive them. We can be awfully hard on ourselves. But failing is part of trying and searching for the right answers. Failing is what occasionally happens when we strive for a better life, when we seek change or adventure. Even the smallest movement will help us reduce pain more than doing nothing. Through experimentation we discover unexpected lessons that aid us in life and in fighting our pain. As long as you keep moving and keep trying, you are on the right path. Your perspective will matter in how you move ahead. The frustration of your pain, the part of you that feels broken, can become your strength.

Current inability does not make anyone a failure. You haven't failed until you have given up. Until then, you are learning. The body learns and can be reprogrammed. Experiences are not isolated. Failing the task at hand doesn't mean that nothing has been gained along the way. It is precisely that failing that will get you to the next step. What is your vision of your life with less pain? Allow yourself to imagine where you are headed. Then set attainable goals you can meet along the way. One goal can be finding a practitioner to guide you. Couple your vision with a strategy of concrete plans and you are on your way to success.

Tools in Your Tool Belt

Now that you have a better understanding of pain, here are some immediate steps you can take to start taking control over your pain.

- **Start Paying Attention.** Assess the pain. Try to pinpoint where you are feeling it. Notice if anything seems to aggravate it: a long car ride, sitting for a while, your bed, extra stress. How would you categorize your discomfort on a pain scale of one to ten? Does the level change throughout the day, week, month, or according to the weather? Remember to notice when you feel good too. Consider recording the answer to all these questions in a journal or on your phone.

- **Breathe.** Breathing is an underutilized tool that allows us to chill out. When our nerves are screaming at us, they need to relax. Pain can create stress and puts our body in fight-or-flight mode. We actually work against ourselves. Taking time to calm ourselves quiets the mind, relaxes the body, fuels the muscles, and is endlessly beneficial. We take breathing for granted, but it is one way for you to regain control.

- **Massage.** You can gently apply pressure or massage the area in pain. If it feels too intense, massage around the area that hurts. Since everything is connected, massaging near the direct site of pain still reduces scar tissue and improves the injured area. Seeing a massage therapist is an added bonus if it is an option for you.

- **Apply Ice or Rubs.** Find a muscle rub you like and apply it before bed. Ice two to three times per day for 15 or 20 minutes. Don't have 15 minutes? Do what you can. Ice is almost never a bad option. You can purchase ice packs that attach to you so that you can ice on the go. If ice seems to aggravate your symptoms, stay away from ice for now. Reevaluate later.

- **Move.** If we do not move, pain worsens. Even the subtlest movement is never worthless, so start with micro-movements. The body does not require all or nothing. Find whatever subtle movement you can do. Play with movements that cause no pain or minimal pain (never going higher than a three on your pain scale of one to ten). Hopefully, you can find a position or motion that provides relief, but even if that doesn't happen right away, continue moving through whatever range you have retained. When the body feels good, it's easy to take basic movements for granted. Yet, if you become paralyzed and then one day were able to wiggle a finger, you would be overcome with joy. Allow yourself to be thrilled by movements that do not hurt, no matter how minimal. Seek pleasure in what you are capable of today.

- **Control What You Can.** You may not be able to stop the pain with a nose wiggle like Samantha Stephens on *Bewitched,* but you can change your diet, your level of exercise, and some of the ergonomics of your furniture. You need not purchase all new furniture. If you are the only one with back pain in your family, consider getting one new seat for the dining room table. Make sure the seat is flat, not curved or indented for your butt. Make sure the section your legs go over is square, not round. Try sitting with the corner between your legs instead of with your legs off the edge.

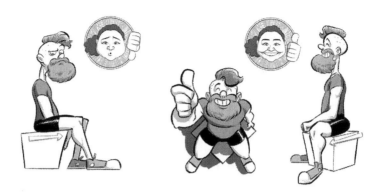

Experiment with everything you can. Sometimes the answer is simple. It is possible that one pair of shoes is causing your plantar fasciitis. We cannot change our genes and often we cannot change our jobs, but we can alter how each one influences our body.

- **Keep Moving.** From small moves, progress to bigger and bigger moves. Check out the chapters in this book with specific exercises for different types of chronic pain. Mark the exercises that feel the best in your body or that you find give you the most relief and best results. You do have to persevere through pain, but pain does not respond to pain. You don't have to push yourself to a point of agony. It's better to keep exploring where in your body you can move and what you can move that doesn't make you cringe. Our bodies are more likely to respond positively if we treat them with kindness. The Golden Rule works even when we are talking about the relationship with our own physique.

- **Relax.** I know, it is the worst thing you can tell someone. You may be shooting me the evil eye right now, but allowing yourself to relax or catching yourself in moments where you can release tension will be helpful. It links back to the first point of assessing and noticing the pain. When we ache, we tend to contract and tense. We brace to protect ourselves. That tension begets more tension. Part of relaxing can be simply noticing when and where your body gets tense and trying to relax unnecessarily engaged muscles. If you are a supporter of meditation, try it. This is not a skill I have, but meditation is incredibly beneficial.

Changing the Brain on Pain

Pain can get us stuck in a rut. When my little brother was a child, he would only eat beige food: pasta with butter, chicken fingers, vanilla ice cream, and Entenmann's Pop'ems (not the chocolate ones) were his entire eating repertoire. Today, he's open to trying most foods and has a considerably more varied palate, but I still presume he'll only want pasta. The brain can get wired to remember something from years ago, no matter how many times we have seen a change. Similarly, something I do all the time—like driving—might suddenly cause me harm one day. Even though the brain has multiple references that driving is typically fine, it is so intent on keeping me safe after an accident that I may be nervous to drive. With physical injuries, our brains can get stuck in the past, harp on one incident and make us think we cannot move forward, or make us afraid to literally move. We need to change the way we think.

This isn't to say that we can simply think ourselves out of any situation. Our minds can change our perspective, but they cannot cure melanoma, dementia, or a slipped disc. If they can, we haven't learned how yet. While the brain is amazing, the body does have a role to play and deserves some of the credit for the good and the bad that happens to us. When you are sick or in pain, it is easy to blame yourself, but it's not helpful. Your brain didn't make you sick. You did not give yourself rheumatoid arthritis, fibromyalgia, or chronic low back pain. You can alter your perspective, but you cannot imagine away what is physically happening in your body.

However, if you keep telling yourself you cannot change, feel better, or make progress, that powerful gray matter has a good chance of stalling you. Just because you haven't been able to improve in the past does not mean you never will be able to in the future. You can start telling yourself you can, even if right now you cannot. Basically, instead of "I can't," consider "I think I can," or "I'm getting there." It's the *Little Engine That Could* tactic. Your mindset determines whether or not you stick to a new plan. Humans are good at rationalizing our way out of tasks we would rather skip.

When you feel stuck, remind yourself that you always have tools in your tool belt. Whether you have learned which tool is right for which project is another story. Trust that with patience and experimentation, you will learn. I know you want the pain to disappear today. Most quick fixes treat the symptom, but do not resolve the problem. Movement can resolve the problem. Movement can heal you.

CHAPTER 2: FITNESS MISCONCEPTIONS THAT HOLD YOU BACK

When it comes to movement, false assumptions wind up being excuses that hold us back and may even contribute to our pain. It is time to debunk some of the myths about movement we have been told our entire lives. Some facts will be a relief and may open up more movement options. Others might be frustrating to learn, because they were too good to be true. Once upon a time, women shoved themselves into vibrating belts and believed they could jiggle off unwanted fat. Nothing we desire comes easily, and no belt is going to burn fat. But when we understand what works and what does not, then we are empowered to better choose movements that work for us.

There is no definitively right or wrong way to move. Sprints, heavy weights, running, bounding, extreme fitness, gentle stretching, sports, Tai Chi—there is a time and a place for all types of movement. That does not mean that all those choices are good for you and your body in this moment. Let's take a look at the more common myths around fitness and how they may be preventing you from moving as much as you should.

I don't have enough time.

This is never really true of anything. We have the time; it's a matter of how we prioritize our time. Most of us have the ability to reorganize our schedule. If you get together with friends, you could ask to go for a walk instead of meeting up for food or coffee. If you sit on the couch in front of a TV, you could get up and march in place. If your child has after-school sports, you can walk the track while they do their activity. Break up movements, such as walking for 15 minutes on your lunch break with gentle stretching for 15 minutes right before bed. Or change how you think about exercise. If you truly can't imagine fitting in 30 minutes of traditional exercise, you can find ways to play with the body throughout the day. It counts. Any movement you can incorporate into your day is a place to start. It's a movement hack. You could do simple exercises while you pump gas or stand and pace while on a phone call. If you go to the mall, a doctor's office, or work, park farther away so you walk longer and take stairs instead of the escalator or elevator. Get creative in ways you can **TAKE MORE STEPS** during the day.

You may not have to set aside 10 or 30 minutes each day to reach your desired fitness level.[13] All the little short bursts you fit in throughout the day can add up to 30 minutes as long as you reach

---

13 Duke University School of Medicine, "Duke-Led Study Finds that Moderate-to-Vigorous Workouts Reduce Mortality," Duke University Health System, March 22, 2018, https://medicine.duke.edu/medicinenews/duke-led-study-finds-moderate-vigorous-workouts-reduce-mortality.

a level of moderate exercise (meaning you have exerted yourself enough that you find it difficult to carry on a conversation). These short bursts may be enough to increase lifespan and reduce disease. You can make changes that don't require adding an hour of exercise. Start by altering small behaviors every day and build from there.

I'm too tired and feel fatigued.

Sometimes we do require rest, and it is okay to allow ourselves to have a break. Sleep enables us to heal and is especially important when we are injured. But we need to ask: am I tired and need a break, or am I just looking for an excuse? Sometimes getting started is the hardest part, and once we are moving, it isn't as bad as we expected. Plus, exercise helps us sleep better and produces an energy boost during our day, so you have less of an urge to reach for a cup of coffee or a sugary treat during the midday slump at work.

For improved sleep, stick with an exercise routine. The results may not be immediate in helping you gets some shut eye. Thirty minutes of exercise three times per week has been shown to improve sleep in women with insomnia after 16 weeks. It's worth the wait. Many of the study participants gained an extra 1.25 hours of sleep per night.[14] Sleep and exercise share a cyclical relationship. The more sleep we get, the more likely we are to exercise and for a longer period. With more sleep, exercise feels better. If you are really tired, try a short walk or a few minutes of stretching. It may not be the moderate aerobic exercise that will eventually help you sleep, but it is still movement that you can feel good about.

---

14 Kelly Glazer Baron et al., "Exercise to Improve Sleep in Insomnia: Exploration of the Bidirectional Effects." *Journal of Clinical Sleep Medicine* 9, no. 8 (2013): 819–24. http://dx.doi.org/10.5664/jcsm.2930.

Go big or go home.

Many people presume that exercise is only beneficial if it's intense, like doing intervals or a boot camp class. Research on the benefits of high intensity interval training seems to encourage that belief. Intense workouts can be advantageous, and if you enjoy that kind of movement, and it is a safe activity for your fitness level, continue having fun in challenging classes. But if crazy jumping workouts and push-ups-until-you-collapse turns you off, don't let it hold you back. When it comes to movement, harder isn't better.

A Danish study lead by Jacob Marott tracked over 1,000 runners for 12 years and revealed a clear bell curve for running speed, duration, and cardiovascular benefit.[15] Runners who ran an average of 15 miles per week and maintained roughly a 10-minute-per-mile pace experienced major cardiovascular benefits and added about six years to their lives. Runners who ran more miles at a faster pace, however, actually demonstrated diminished cardiovascular gains. Their workload was too challenging for the heart, reducing the potential gain of a moderate run. They might as well have been couch potatoes, because they earned zero cardiovascular benefit.

If you love running fast, you don't have to stop. There could be other benefits outside of cardiovascular health. You may find stress relief or joy in a sprint. The point is this: if you think that to achieve any positive gain you have to work harder or faster, you absolutely do not. You get to be the judge of what vigorous means, because it's different for everyone. One woman's brisk walk is another man's saunter, possibly providing the same benefit. Moderate exercise, where you are winded but can catch

---

15 Kathleen Doheny, "Here's How Much Running Is Healthiest for You, According to One Study," *Health*, February 2, 2015.

your breath enough to talk, is believed to be a healthy level for new exercisers. You need to find the movement that is right for you at this moment.

When in pain, any movement is beneficial and better than nothing. Subtle, micro-movements are optimal and make a big impact long term. As pain decreases, the size of a movement will increase. You can also move parts of your body that aren't in pain. If your neck aches, can you move your shoulder pain-free? Remind your body that it can move. That moveable part will trickle toward the stiff area. If you don't move it, the stiff portion spreads. Working our way out of pain comes through subtlety. Never underestimate what your body is gaining or how it is changing from a mini-move. Big moves require big muscles. Small moves require control over much smaller muscles deep inside, and it is from this place that our true stability and strength originate. There have been multiple, although often small, studies that suggest small movements can help reduce pain. A UCLA study of children and young adults with chronic pain and rheumatoid arthritis found reduced levels of pain after practicing Iyengar yoga, which emphasizes proper alignment and incorporates modified poses that keep movements small and gentle. A review of multiple studies on tai chi demonstrated that this ancient Chinese practice can help reduce pain and stiffness for people with osteoarthritis.[16] Gentle, small movements can make a big difference in quality of life. Moving simply because it feels good to your body is beneficial, and you do not always, or ever, have to be in burnout mode to see results. Find the level you love.

---

16 Yi-Wen Chen et al., "The Effect of Tai Chi on Four Chronic Conditions—Cancer, Osteoarthritis, Heart Failure and Chronic Obstructive Pulmonary Disease: A Systematic Review and Meta-Analyses," *British Journal of Sports Medicine* 50, no. 7 (2016): 397–407, https://bjsm.bmj.com/content/50/7/397.info.

Trust your instincts. Because our culture encourages pushing too hard, too fast, we tend to either reach beyond our current limit, which leads to setbacks, or we hold ourselves back by presuming what we do is not enough. It is okay to start moving five to ten minutes per day for five days a week. All movement counts. Generally, once you get started, you'll extend your activity time and will learn the pace at which your body is ready to move. If you are feeling pain or notice an ache a day later, ease up next time. Your muscles make progress faster than your tendons, ligaments, and fascia. So, if you work at your muscles' pace, other parts of your body may be struggling to keep up. Tendons, ligaments, and other soft tissue can take six months to two years to make the same changes that happen in your muscles in a few weeks. It's important to be attentive to how the whole body—mind, fascia, nerves—reacts to adding exercise. Find the pace and level of exercises that challenge you but don't push you too far (and hopefully brings you some enjoyment, too!). Most importantly, find a way to keep moving.

Exercise has to hurt or there is no benefit.

"No pain, no gain" is a fallacy that has made too many people hate moving for too long. We can blame Jane Fonda for popularizing the tagline in her aerobics workouts from the '80s, but it was really Ben Franklin who wrote it first in *Poor Richard's Almanac*. "There are no gains without pains" doesn't roll off the tongue in quite the same way when filming a snappy, upbeat workout video where every breath counts. In terms of exercise, the opposite is true. Pain is a signal to stop. Those who don't listen wind up injured. If your workout causes an injury or you need Ibuprofen to get through it, it is not the workout for you.

It's important to differentiate between types of pain in movement. "My quads (front of your thighs) feel sore while I'm doing squats" is a different sensation than "Gee, my knees are cracking, and there's a sharp pain every time I squat." We need to learn to tell the difference between "good" and "bad" pain, and then listen to those signals from the body while they are still whispers. When we listen, we learn to take breaks to minimize our potential for injury. When our muscles are fatigued, but we keep pushing, we risk injuring joints and soft tissue, like tendons. We must heed their warning when muscles communicate that they are tired or we can end up hurting ourselves. Feeling your back twinge, your neck ache, or your wrists throb is a "bad" hurt that you should never work through. When you feel and push through pain, you are training your body to view pain as an acceptable occurrence during movement. Who would want to move if agony was the end result? When you move to increase strength, cardio, and overall health, strive for challenging but manageable maneuvers.

Sometimes I have clients tell me that they didn't feel sore after a class, and they want to feel that post-workout ache. It is an uphill battle to try to unconvince people of an idea we learned as children. You do not have to feel sore after a workout for it to have been effective. Yet, we believe that if we aren't grunting, dripping with sweat, and falling to the floor in exhaustion, that we haven't done enough. If you are that sore after a workout, the little muscles that stabilize you have probably been completely bypassed. And that pain may diminish the benefits of tomorrow's workout. Delayed Onset Muscle Soreness (DOMS), that ache in your muscles somewhere between 24 and 48 hours after exercising, is unnecessary. You go to sit down, walk up a flight of stairs, or squat over the toilet and realize you have muscles you have been taking for granted. If you love the feeling of DOMS, it won't become a disincentive to move. But if you don't like that feeling and never want to feel it, know that an effective workout does not require sore muscles or pain.[17] Some muscles in the body

---

17 Brad J. Schoenfeld and Bret Contreras, "Is Postexercise Muscle Soreness a Valid Indicator of Muscular Adaptations?" *Strength and Conditioning Journal* 35, no. 5 (Oct 2013): 16–21, https://doi.org/10.1519/SSC.0b013e3182a61820.

experience more DOMS than others. Some people genetically experience the sensation of DOMS more than others without it serving as an accurate indicator of how challenging the workout was. Without that delayed fatigue, you will still build strength and progress. Not pushing until your legs shake does not mean you are a slacker. Unless you are a student athlete, Olympian, or training to be the next American Ninja Warrior (which would be awesome), there's no need to feel sore after a workout in order for it to have been productive. It's a fallacy that has besieged our love of movement for decades. Our new motto should be: "no pain, no pain." Movement is the best way to escape our pain. All movement counts, and your body is grateful. Stop presuming that if you do not feel sore, there is no point. Begin slowly. You can always build up.

We need to check our egos at the door when we start to move. Learning what level we can work at is an experiment. It changes year-to-year, day-to-day, and class-to-class. What is your goal? If you want to be an Olympic skater, your workout routine will be different than if you want to be able to hike Mt. Washington or play with your children or always be able to get down to and up from the floor. Pick your target and find the moves that help you attain that objective.

I have bad knees or a bad [insert name of body part here].

If anyone tells you that a particular movement—squatting, reaching overhead, twisting—is bad for you, ask them how you are going to do the actual movement in life in order to function. You do a squat to get in and out of a chair, the car, and to sit on the toilet. Your arm needs to go overhead to grab a dish out of the cupboard. You have to twist to look at your blind spot when driving. No movement should be permanently off the table. Exercises may need to be modified for a time, but the end goal should be functional movement required of you in normal life. People with joint replacements might have particular limitations, but still need to maintain as much mobility as possible. The worst scenario is to stop moving and allow the restriction to spread elsewhere in the body.

We are told running is bad for our joints and that squats are bad for our knees. It's not true. Our bodies were made to be able to run. That doesn't mean they were meant to run for eight hours without stopping or to run 26.2 miles at a time. But our bones grow and respond to the stress we place on them.[18] That means running, weight lifting, and high intensity workouts can all be positive for bone health. Nothing about those activities is inherently bad for us. Injuries, skill level, form, strength, and flexibility all work together to determine which option is best for any individual's bones and body. Maintaining good form right now for you might mean performing fewer repetitions, finding subtle weight shifts that help you execute a movement without pain, or smaller ranges of motion. You might benefit from someone teaching you proper form that will be less taxing on joints or tendons if you can't find a way that doesn't cause pain on your own.

Our bodies are versatile and adaptable. They can learn and relearn new patterns. If movement hurts, you never want to force it, but you need to learn how to do every movement required for an increased quality of life. When someone tells you that you should not do a particular movement, question them and seek another opinion. There is almost no injury that can't be improved by movement. Move, while listening to the feedback from your body, and you will feel better. If you've ever pulled your back,

18 19th century anatomist, Julius Wolff in Wolff's Law

you know this to be true. Lie still, and it gets worse. While you can't run a marathon with a pulled back, you absolutely can and should move. Immobilization post injury or after certain surgeries is worse than appropriate early mobilization.[19] The type of injury and location in the body may require different needs, but the more we learn, the more the answer becomes: KEEP MOVING.

You need someone to tell you what to do.

I love working with clients, and I enjoy attending a good fitness class for the energy and social aspect. If time or money is an issue, you don't like group classes, or no classes in your area fit your schedule, you have other choices. You can download free exercise videos, subscribe to online classes through services like YogaGlo, John Garey TV, or find ways to create your own movement. One of Joe Pilates's goals was to create a movement sequence that people could do on their own, every day.

Pilates elders are the men and women who trained under Joe Pilates and continued teaching into their 80s and 90s, and every elder I've trained with has encouraged me to be creative in movement. As an adult, crafting our own moves can be intimidating, which is sad. For a species dependent on movement, we are cautious and hesitant, and constantly second guess ourselves because somewhere along the line we were trained to believe a movement was right or wrong, but that is an erroneous concept. No movement is wrong or right. Movement doesn't

---

19 Pekka Kannus, "Immobilization or Early Mobilization After an Acute Soft-Tissue Injury?" The Physician and Sportsmedicine 28, no. 3 (Jun 2015): 55–63, https://doi.org/10.3810/psm.2000.03.775; A. C. Cook et al., "Early Mobilization Following Carpal Tunnel Release. A Prospective Randomized Study," Journal of Hand Surgery 20, no. 2 (1995): 228–30, https://doi.org/10.1016/S0266-7681(05)80057-9; C. E. Nash et al., "Injured Limbs Recover Better with Early Mobilization and Functional Bracing Than with Cast Immoblization," The Journal of Bone & Joint Surgery 87, no. 5 (2005): 1167, https://doi.org/10.2106/JBJS.8705.ebo3.

have to be ordered and controlled. Understanding proper form will get you more out of an exercise and encourage healing, but if a movement feels glorious in your body, enjoy it. Seek out better, more efficient, fun, feel-good moves that encourage a return to movement.

One time, I worked with an elder who told me to make up an exercise on a piece of equipment called the ladder barrel, which looks like a large hump attached to a short ladder about three feet away from the hump. I put myself in one position, laying over the barrel on my back in a blissful backbend. "That's nothing new," she said. "Someone has done that before." I tried again with another move that lacked creativity. I repeated unoriginal moves a couple of times with the same unimpressed response, and then I contorted myself into a miserable, precarious position, sort of upside down as if in an awkward, dangerous, aerial game of Twister. She looked at me quizzically and said, "That looks so uncomfortable. Why would you pick that position?" I created it out of desperation to finally have her say she approved of my creation. And now I was stuck there and had to figure out how to get my feet back on solid ground without looking like an incompetent student of movement. You don't need to make up original moves. You can move any way that feels good.

Remember when you were a teenager, and you'd turn on music and dance in your room like no one was watching? (Maybe this is just girls. Maybe it's just me.) This week, try dancing to a song of your choice. By the end, if you aren't smiling or don't feel good, you'll have wasted two minutes at worst. When I was a child, my mom and I listened to show tunes and made up dances to go with them. "A Chorus Line" was a favorite, and Jimmy Durante's "Make Someone Happy" was another good choice. We'd go over it and over it as if we were rehearsing for a performance. We were exercising, and neither one of us had any idea. It is one of many fond memories of time with my mother.

We should always stretch before exercise.

I love stretching and recommend it in certain situations, but if you hate it, you have other options that might yield the same results. Years ago, I was at the gym and saw a woman stretching. She looked so graceful and made the stretches look effortless. I've always felt tight in my body and wished I could stretch as far as she could reach. I mentioned it, saying, "I wish I was as flexible as you." She responded, "Oh, I wish I was as strong as you." I remember being shocked that someone so comfortably contorted would want to step into my body. Together we'd be a winning combination. Humans need both strength and flexibility.

We anatomically created beginnings and ends for muscles and tendons, when in reality everything is connected and flows or intertwines into the next part. When you picture stretching a muscle, recognize the muscle can only get so long. A muscle becomes a tendon, which connects to a bone. Each individual part only has so much range of motion. If you have a tight muscle, you cannot unhook the beginning and pin it higher up to actually lengthen it. There is only so much wiggle room to play with when it comes to stretching. If a muscle is tight and we attempt to stretch it beyond where it is ready to lengthen, it is likely that something besides the targeted muscle, like a tendon, is going to stretch. No part of our body can act in isolation. When we stretch, we need to be sure we are stretching the muscle to a point that doesn't strain the body. Many people who hate stretching follow the no pain, no gain rule and try to stretch more than is necessary for results. It hurts, they hate it, and they stop doing it.

Helene Langevin's research revealed that stretching might impact our fascia (connective tissue touching everything in the body) by reducing inflammation, therefore reducing pain.[20] But, as is the theme of this book, to relieve pain, you don't need to work to the point of pain. For example, you don't need to hold a stretch until you are shaking. That's not relaxing. Agonizing stretches are an attempt to whip your body into submission. You basically force a stretch and put a muscle into the equivalent of fight-or-fight mode. The muscles think (yes, I can tell what muscles are thinking), "Oh no! I'm stretched to my limit! I can't do my job. I better tense and hold onto the structure for dear life." That muscle isn't going to find ease. If you want stretching to have any chance of working for you, you need to go to a place where you feel a stretch, pause, and try to relax. It is generally accepted that 30 seconds is the magic number where you receive maximum benefit from that stretch.

If you still aren't sold on the idea of stretching, foam rolling might be an option to "stretch" you. If rolling your muscles and tendons on a firm piece of foam feels good and doesn't bring a tear to your eye, you might be able to relax muscles with it. A small study on college athletes found that foam rolling reduced post-workout fatigue.[21] Additional research indicates it increases flexibility in the short term and possibly long term when done regularly.[22] However, if it causes pain, cease and desist. We must eliminate the mindset that we should push ourselves to pain to improve anything. Why would the body ever be on our side if we are constantly hurting it? We need to rebuild trust with our own body.

---

20 Professor in Residence of Medicine at Harvard Medical School and Neurology, Orthopedics and Rehabilitation at the University of Vermont College of Medicine, and Director of the Osher Center for Integrative Medicine Harvard Medical School and Brigham and Women's Hospital.

21 Kellie C. Healey et al.,"The Effects of Myofascial Release with Foam Rolling on Performance," *Journal of Strength and Conditioning Research* 28, no. 1, (Jan 2014): 61–68, https://doi.org/10.1519/JSC.0b013e3182956569.

22 Sonja Ristevski, "Do Foam Rollers Actually Work? A Review of the Evidence," Healthy But Smart, updated May 3, 2018, https://healthybutsmart.com/foam-rollers/.

Whatever you do, don't stretch before an intense workout or weight lifting. It's been known for probably a decade now that there is no proven gain and that in fact you might have diminished returns. In trying to lengthen muscles before you need them to work, you are actually weakening and then burdening them. Stretch after your workout when muscles are warm to reduce injuries. Warm-ups need to be dynamic. Very small, limited studies show foam rolling may help warm the body. Bottom line: stretch gently and within a safe range for you or consider foam rolling if you find it more fun than stretching.

Sit-ups strengthen your abs.

Would it be a relief if I told you that you never had to do another sit-up again? Those fast-paced curls are the old-school exercise of the American fitness test ("Let's see how many sit-ups all these kids can crank out in one minute!"). For years, it has not seemed to matter that the standard sit-up often does not use abdominal muscles. Instead, they regularly strain hip flexors and put unnecessary pressure on the back. In our youth, many of us get away with bad form on a sit-up, but over time it trains us to use faulty patterns.

The *psoas* is one of your hip flexors that connects to all of your lumbar (low back) vertebrae. When you race through a series of sit-ups, ultimately the psoas gets involved, tugging on your lower back and creating strain. Even the military is now looking to remove sit-ups from its standard fitness testing and replace them with planks, which target the abs more effectively. The truth is that either exercise done with poor form can aggravate the back.

Our end goal is not simply completing the task at hand. Who cares if you held a sloppy plank for two minutes or raced through 100 sit-ups in a set time. The goal should be controlled, functional, safe movement. In movement, we need to discover where we have strength, whether something stiff and inflexible is holding us back, and how to move from a point of control. If I complete a sit-up and get to the top but have put my back at risk and haven't used my muscles to their best ability, what have I gained? It looks like I can do it, but so what? You can do sit-ups for five minutes and get nothing out of it. Or, you can do a 15-second plank and have improved your body. You have to trust that less can be more and commit to quality over quantity.

Your core means your abdominals.

You've probably heard the term *core*. It's a common buzz word, and most people think core and picture their abs. The core actually includes the abs, the glutes (butt muscles), the back muscles, and the shoulder girdle (basically your entire trunk). You need a strong, solid, yet pliable frame for your limbs to move and pull on. When you move, you should feel stability and strength throughout your core. It's all connected. Your arm is a lot more useful when you see it as an extension of your core. You have strength from your ribs, waist, and hips to throw a ball, swing a golf club, or lift a heavy bag. The deepest muscles of the core (the pelvic floor, transversus abdominis, and multifidus) are intricately linked to stress reductions, good posture, and reduced chronic back pain.

For core stability you need to do ab exercises, back exercises, butt exercises, and shoulder exercises. Many of us, especially if we sit at a desk and tend to slouch forward, create short abdominal muscles. More sit-ups or crunches may not be best for strengthening the core. Our ab-centric attitudes may be limiting us. It's not all or nothing. Our body requires a combination of movement. For a healthy core, we need to bend forward, bend back, twist, and bend side to side. Variety is vital.

It's really nutrition that is important.

Ugh! This one really bothers me. I've read articles alluding to the fact that it is more important to eat right than to exercise. Can't both be important to our health and well-being? According to a 2015 *New York Times* article, exercise increases weight gain because it makes you want to eat more.[23] The not-so-hidden message there is to stop exercising, but that is really misleading information.

This presumptuously assumes we only exercise to lose weight. For everything else the body needs—basic wellness, cardiovascular health, flexibility, mobile joints—you absolutely must move. Even if it were all about losing weight, exercise matters. Increase activity and burn more calories, and you should lose weight. But, exercise makes you hungry and then you eat more. If you eat more and do not make healthy food choices, of course, that will negate your calorie burn from the workout. Anyone who suggests you should not move is doing you perhaps the greatest disservice of your life. Read between the lines when you are drawn in by snazzy headlines.

While people can lose weight by altering their diet and cutting calories, it is exercise that often makes people feel better about their bodies. Anecdotally, people will tell me, "I started doing Pilates, and now I feel taller" or "Since I started walking, my abs and body feel tighter." Movement is imperative to health.

Exercise is boring.

If you have never found a type of movement you like, try something else. If you get bored easily, make sure you have a

---

23 Aaron E. Carroll, "To Lose Weight, Eating Less Is Far More Important Than Exercising More," *The New York Times*, June 15, 2015.

different exercise plan for each day of the week. You don't have to do the same thing every day. In fact, variation is better for your body. Walk, run, or take a class with a buddy so you can socialize while you work out. Put on your favorite TV program, grab a timer, and pick any move, doing a move for one minute and then switching. Keep rotating through moves until your TV show is over. Incorporate gamification, using technology like the Wii, or FitBit or another tracker. Move for points. Create competition if that's your thing. If you have to move (which you do) and you are resistant to it, make it a game.

A few years ago, I was in San Antonio, Texas with my boyfriend and favorite travel companion, Matt. Across from the Alamo, we stumbled across a laser game where your mission (should you choose to accept it) is to crawl, scamper, plank, and contort your body to finagle your way through a room of lasers. You must get from one side to the other without ever touching any lasers with your body. Even your ponytail can't meet a red line puncturing the room (becoming self-aware of your hair can be a challenge, especially for someone who was raised in the 80s). You feel like you're in *Mission Impossible*. It's delightful in every way. Matt and I played over and over for 90 minutes without even noticing the time was passing. Games can be exercise, and exercise can be fun. I didn't realize I was getting a workout until I noticed I was sweating. The following day when I was sore all over, particularly in my shoulders, it struck me: I was fooled into a fabulous workout, and I was oblivious at the time.

Movement is vital to life. You must find a way to make the task fun. Perhaps it starts by no longer associating it with exercise, but instead spending time outdoors lubricating your joints while walking with a friend. There is no wrong answer to the movement you choose. Hiking, kayaking, running, cycling, aerobics, Pilates, or dancing—if the movement gives you joy, it is the move for you. Try not to let expectations thwart your efforts. Don't always worry about if it is "right" or "perfect." Allow yourself to move and laugh at yourself when you look silly.

My gear matters.

Better shoes or tools can help, but they aren't required to get moving. You can get creative with items you have at home. You can use soup cans as weights or an old belt or towel to help you stretch a tight muscle. You can do bicep curls with filled grocery bags as you walk in the house. Stairs can become an exercise machine. Tennis balls can provide a gentle massage. A partially-filled, frozen water bottle can be used to ice the body. My grandfather used to sew sand into old squares of cloth to make bean bags that he used as leg weights. Walking should not require more than a pair of sneakers. Get creative and know that having the perfect outfit or the nicest set of equipment isn't required to get moving. If having something new motivates you, use it as a tool. You can always treat yourself to new attire if you met your exercise goals that month.

CHAPTER 3: YOU ARE NOT ALONE IN THIS

The most important thing to remember as you embark on this journey is that you are not alone, even if sometimes it feels that way. Over 100 million Americans are tormented by chronic pain. That's about one out of every three people. In the United States, you could combine everyone who has cancer, heart disease, and diabetes and there would be 40 million fewer people affected by those conditions than those suffering from pain. Pain is our most prevalent medical condition and costs society $560 to $635 billion annually.[24] Globally, it's estimated that 1.5 billion, or roughly 20 percent of the population, are experiencing chronic pain.[25]

---

24 Darrell J. Gaskin and Patrick Richard, "The Economic Costs of Pain in the United States," *The Journal of Pain* 13, no. 8 (Aug 2012): 715–724, https://doi.org/10.1016/j.jpain.2012.03.009.

25 Rolf-Detlef Treede et al., "A Classification of Chronic Pain for *ICD-11*," *Pain* 156, no. 6 (Jun 2015): 1003–7, http://doi.org/10.1097/j.pain.0000000000000160.

You may feel judged. You may judge yourself. You look at that other guy with back pain, and he seems to push through so much more than you do. But no two people feel anything exactly the same. Your bodies are not the same, your injuries are not the same, and your pains are not the same. When you compare, it is never a fair comparison. Ultimately, only *you* know what *you* feel. Pain is complicated. Figuring out what works may pose potential challenges, but there is an answer.

As important as it is to find something that works for your pain, it is equally important to be cautious about some of the solutions offered out there, particularly pain medication. While there is a time and a place when pain medication can be helpful, we have also learned about the dangers of dependence. Over 20,000 Americans died from an overdose of opioids in 2015, and that doesn't include the over 10,000 heroin addicts who died from overdose. [26] As a society, we have a problem. People are in pain and are prescribed medication that needs to be taken very carefully. Unfortunately, that medication doesn't have many studies supporting long-term effectiveness, but it does cause addiction and can lead to death. While the prevalence is unknown, people on opioids sometimes develop opioid-induced hyperalgesia. That's a hefty name for increased pain sensations. Nearly two million people in the United States have a substance abuse issue that involves prescription painkillers.[27] We have a problem, and we are medicating it, which is creating even more dangerous problems. We must look to other ways to resolve physical pain. When Prince died, he was taking fentanyl for hip pain, a legal, prescription medication which is up to 50 times more potent than morphine or heroin. That is why you are not

---

26 American Society of Addiction Medicine, "Opioid Addiction 2016 Facts & Figures," Accessed July 2018, https://www.asam.org/docs/default-source/advocacy/opioid-addiction-disease-facts-figures.pdf.
27 American Society of Addiction Medicine, "Opioid Addiction 2016 Facts & Figures."

alone. Even the rich and famous get desperate and caught in a downward spiral when living with chronic pain.

More than half of the nation's daily drug overdose deaths are from heroin and prescription painkillers.[28] There is a misconception that heroin addicts are homeless, mentally ill, sick individuals, not people like us. In truth, many of those who have died are just like us, dealing with an injury and in pain. They were prescribed pills by a trusted doctor, became dependent on them, and then needed an option when the prescription ran out. Not everyone in pain turns to heroin, but let's ensure it does not become your life. Let's get moving, and let exercise be our medicine.

I've been using the word exercise throughout this book, because we all know what it means. But the "E" word has a negative connotation for many people. When you read that word, think of it as interchangeable with movement. Let's redefine exercise to mean *any movement (big or small, fast or slow, challenging or easy, subtle or intense) that enables us to feel, reminds us we are alive, and gets us to our goal.* Movement is not droning, repetitive exercises. Movement is life.

We are about to delve deep into a world of anatomy to discuss muscles, tendons, bones, and nerves. Hopefully after this little lesson, you will fall madly in love with the idea of moving your body. Before your new love affair with movement starts, let's actually move. Try these movements and know that if that is all you do today, it is enough for now. Once you have finished reading through this page of exercises, snap a picture so you can easily refer to them later and do them regularly.

---

28 American Society of Addiction Medicine, "Opioid Addiction 2016 Facts & Figures."

Movement Break: Eight Easy Exercises Everyone Can Do!

There may be a reason someone should not do certain movements, but for the most part, these moves are safe and beneficial for nearly everyone. If you are not typically active, this is a good way to introduce movement. If you are super active, this is a great way to ensure you focus on every part of your body, even the parts you often skip over. Incorporate these eight exercises throughout your day. Recruit friends, family, or coworkers to do them with you. Nothing should hurt when you do these moves, so stop or skip any that hurt. The total series should take fewer than 10 minutes.

The order doesn't matter, but remember the acronym STARTUPS! Try them morning, noon, and night. Do them to your heart's delight. (Uh, oh. I've started rhyming. Definitely time to move...)

Shoulder Lifts:

- Sit or stand with your arms long at your sides.

- Slide your shoulders up by your ears like you are doing a shoulder shrug.

- Lower your shoulders back down.

- Try different variations. Lift and lower with control. Lift and then let them drop like your arms became dead weight. Try lifting one shoulder and lowering the other.

Toe Lifts:

- Ideally stand but sit if that *feels* better to you.

- Without shifting your weight, lift all ten toes off the floor and lower them.

- Repeat 10 times or until you get bored.

Ankle Circles:

- Sit or stand if you desire a little balance challenge.

- Lift one foot off the ground and circle your ankle in both directions.

- Repeat on the other side.

Rib Twists:

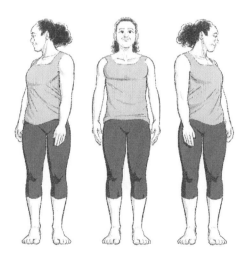

- Sit or stand. Standing makes this more dynamic if you try to twist the ribs while keeping the hips still.

- Rotate your ribs to one side and then to the other.

- Sometimes focus on keeping the hips still. Sometimes let yourself move freely.

- Think of doing the twist, sometimes nice and loose, sometimes more controlled.

Turkey Trots: (for a picture, see page 235)

People with neck injuries, be cautious with this one. If it hurts, stop.

- Sit as tall as you can, lengthening through the spine. Never do this from a slump!

- Try not to let your chin tilt up and down, but keep it level throughout the movement.

- Imagine a turkey strutting. Move your head forward and back.

- When you pull back, it may feel like you are trying to give yourself a double chin.

- Force nothing. Worry less how far forward your head can go (that should be more natural) and pay attention to what it feels like to pull the head back.

Upper Back Motion:

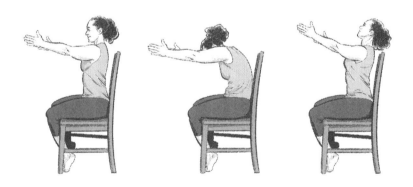

My grandma learned this basic movement when she took belly dancing classes. They called it Tarzan (when you rounded forward) and Jane (when you stuck your breastbone forward).

- Sit or stand. Sitting is a little more comfortable and easier.

- Reach arms straight out in front of you.

- Reach for the wall across the room by spreading your shoulder blades apart (this is called protraction) and rounding forward at the ribs (try not to move the lower back that much).

- Then slide your shoulder blades together (known as retraction), and bring your breastbone forward like you are doing a little backbend of the upper spine.

- Repeat 10 times or keep going if it feels great.

Pelvic Tilts:

See **Pelvic Tilt** picture on page 166

Standing, sitting, or lying down (knees bent and feet on the floor), try them all and have a ball. Whichever position you pick, you are trying to move your pelvis from neutral (a slight arch in your low back) to imprint (a lengthening of the low back).

- Rock your pelvis back and forth.

- Think of tucking your tailbone between your legs like a bad dog and then sticking it out and allowing the lower back to arch.

- Try to make the motion come from your abs, NOT your butt or back.

- Experiment with how big and how small you can make the motion.

- Try to keep your ribs still and legs still.

Standing Hip Circles:

- While standing, open your legs wider than hip distance apart.

- Trace an imaginary hula hoop with your pelvis.

- Reverse.

You just moved every part of your body from top to bottom. Well done, you!

In Good Company

"Exercise and application produce order in our affairs, health of body, cheerfulness of mind, and these make us precious to our friends.... You are not, however, to consider yourself as unemployed while taking exercise. That is necessary for your health, and health is the first of all objects...."

—Thomas Jefferson

When you start moving, you are in good company. When we worked the land, it wasn't as imperative to carve out specific time for movement and call it exercise. We were active. We physically labored all day. My great-grandma never "exercised" a day in her life, but she had muscular arms. Born in 1899, she didn't have electric beaters or mixers so for years all her food was stirred by hand, and she washed clothes without the help of a machine. She was strong, and that musculature was still visible at age 95 even though she had switched over to modern technology by then. The tools that make our lives more convenient are not necessarily good for our health. Riding lawn mowers create another place to sit. Computers trap us at a desk all day. Smartphones tilt our heads down and exhaust our little opposable thumbs.

Prior to all this high tech when our country was forming, the Founding Fathers moved. Thomas Jefferson preferred walking to almost any other movement. He believed "a strong body makes the mind strong" and encouraged taking a 30-minute walk each morning to shake the sleep off and two hours of exercise in the afternoon to break up the day. While Jefferson encouraged increasingly long walks, John Adams, a farmer when living in Massachusetts, regularly walked three to four miles per day.

Before they had medical research to prove it, these men knew the benefits of movement. Adams wrote: "Exercise invigorates and enlivens all the faculties of body and of mind. It arouses our animal spirits, it disperses melancholy. It spreads a gladness and satisfaction over our minds and qualifies us for every sort of business, and every sort of pleasure." He once wrote a letter to Benjamin Franklin stating that "it is a breach of the sixth commandment not to exercise." For context, the sixth commandment forbids us to kill anyone. According to John Adams, if we do not exercise, we are killing ourselves.

Franklin, perhaps surprisingly, is a member of the International Swimming Hall of Fame. Not only was he an avid swimmer, but he invented one of the first fins. While most pictures portray a portly man in his 70s, for most of Franklin's life he was a great proponent of vigorous exercise. He lifted weights and ran up and down stairs, the latter being a movement choice he suggested for anyone short on time. He argued riding horseback was better than taking a carriage and walking was better than riding.

Why does this matter for chronic pain? The voices of these thinkers, these men who led a revolution and started a new country, are reminders that movement is vital to our health. Franklin wrote, "Exercise to prevent diseases, since the cure of them by physics is so precarious." We can take our medical system to task, but it still offers so much that benefits our health. What modern medicine accomplishes for our longevity and quality of life is amazing. But we always have more to learn. When medicine does not work for us or is currently incapable of providing the answer, we can turn to movement. Movement is medicine.

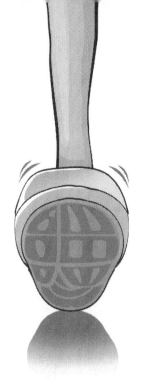

SECTION TWO:
THIS IS YOUR BODY,
AND YOU ONLY
GET ONE!

"Nothing happens until something moves."

—Albert Einstein

When my best friend, Julie, turned 27, in Peter Pan fashion she planned a birthday party for herself filled with elementary school games like Bombardment, kickball, and Spud, a fun game involving running away from balls, chasing balls, pegging balls at people, and had a spanking machine (which looking back seems pretty inappropriate for elementary school).

After eight hours of playing games from our childhood, every party-goer was moaning over an injury. I hurt my hip, which would result in a visit to a physical therapist. Julie's stiff neck permanently connected her right ear to her right shoulder for days and required massage and physical therapy. Matt hurt his back, a previous injury that within a year would require a visit to a physical therapist, and another friend injured his knee. I don't know for sure how everyone felt when they awoke the next morning, but I suspect people were feeling muscles and joints they had spent their entire lives trying to ignore.

Clearly, we were not as young as we felt or as young as we imagined, and playing elementary school games seemed to have the reverse effect from what was desired. Instead of feeling young, we felt really, really old. Pain makes you feel ancient. Joe Pilates wrote, "If your spine is inflexibly stiff at 30, you are old. If it is completely flexible at 60, you are young." No matter how old we are, when our back hurts, we feel 90. How we feel matters more than what age we are.

We played these games for an entire workday and pushed through some of the pain in an effort to convince ourselves that we were still young, a choice that would, in fact, make us appear a bit infantile. Alcohol was involved, restricting sensible choices. By the end of the day, people were reaching into the cooler not for cans of beer but for handfuls of ice to ease the aches and pains. Discovering that a game called Spud could knock us back for a week did not help us find the glorious days of youth we were seeking. Most of the injuries stemmed from incidents earlier in our lives, which reminds us that aging is only part of the pain problem.

Once you have been injured, daily life and regular activities may sometimes aggravate that injury. Ever since that day at the trampoline park, my neck gets irritated when I ride a bike. But you can learn movement tools that help reduce the chances of old injuries rearing their ugly heads. The right tools can help you get back on track faster if the pain ever returns. Knowing that I have been able to get myself out of pain in the past helps me get less tense about current pain. I remind myself whenever I feel pain that in my previous experiences I have always found my way out of pain, even if it has taken a long time. That thought is a comfort. But some people have been in pain so long, it feels impossible to remember a time without it. Or, not having found your way out of pain yet, you are unsure whether you can.

As we age, every part of us is constantly changing. Workouts get harder, cells die, full-time jobs and kids get in the way of fitness routines, and pain makes us want to crawl into bed. No part of life is an excuse to skip exercise. Stop moving, and we create immobility. Finding a safe way to move will keep us younger longer. When we hurt, we have to get back up and keep moving. The art of movement is a balancing act. We need to listen to the body and stop when it tells us to, but we should never stop moving altogether. Everything in moderation, even moderation. We can move too much and get hurt, but if we do not move at all, we are destined to a life of pain. We each need to learn the balance for ourselves. In our ever-changing bodies, that can take a lifetime to learn. But it is that constant change that creates opportunity.

CHAPTER 4: HOW YOUR BODY WORKS

Your body is a tool, and you need to care for it to get the most out of it. Comprehending basic concepts of how the body works together and a general understanding of your anatomy will enable you to find better help, whether searching the internet for answers or advocating for yourself at the doctor's office. Learning basic concepts of the body is like learning the fundamental parts of your car before you take it to the mechanic. Knowledge gives you some clout. If you don't have a baseline understanding of how you are put together and move, when you are in pain, you will be stuck in a drain hole of torture. Knowing more about your body is empowering.

Let's start with a short anatomy review and then discuss pain science. A review of multiple studies has shown that providing people suffering from musculoskeletal pain with a basic understanding about pain neuroscience education—basically understanding how pain works in their bodies—and dialoguing about what they feel in their bodies helps them reduce pain catastrophizing, feel safer about moving more, feel encouraged to use healthcare providers, and create an overall improved attitude toward pain.[29]

But before we explain how pain works, we need to understand how the body works. People usually start learning about anatomy in high school, but it should be taught even earlier. We should learn our muscles like we learn our letters and should grow up knowing how the body functions. Fifth graders should be able to rattle off their muscles and bones in a catchy song. If you worked hard to skip anatomy class in high school, don't worry. I will try to make this painless. Think of this section like anatomy CliffsNotes.

When we understand how a movement will benefit us, we are more likely to do it and get more from that movement. If you are told to do butt exercises to improve your back and you understand why engaging the butt helps, you are more likely to do the exercises. If the explanation seems nonsensical, you are going to question whether it is worth your time. After all, what does your butt have to do with your back? (We will get to that later.)

If you already think you have a pretty keen understanding of anatomy, consider reading this anyway. There has been a lot of recent research that has altered conventional understanding of how we think about movement and our bodies. Some of the information below may still change, but if we continue with our old concepts of movement, they can hold us back. New insights mean new possibilities. When it comes to movement, there is the old paradigm where each individual muscle and bone has a

---

29 Adriaan Louw et al., "The Efficacy of Pain Neuroscience Education on Musculoskeletal Pain: A Systematic Review of the Literature," *Physiotherapy Theory and Practice* 32, no. 5 (2016): 332–35, https://doi.org/10.1080/09593985.2016.1194 646.

specific role; this muscle moves this part and that muscle moves that part. In the new paradigm, everything is connected and affects everything else. It suggests that, since every movement influences every part, we should stop thinking about individual muscles as specific movers. Both concepts can be beneficial when it comes to movement, so the old ideas are not out-of-date.

It is difficult to understand how interconnected everything is when we cannot break it down into separate moving parts. Think of the body as a team sport. Each player is distinct and has a role, but how they all interact together ultimately determines how the entire team performs. A goalie is unlikely to ever score a goal, because that's not what a goalie is supposed to do, just like flaring our nostrils probably will not make our back pain disappear and flexing our calf is not going to turn our head to look for oncoming traffic. But if that goalie does not do her job efficiently and effectively, or worse if the goalie passed out, the whole team suffers. Everyone feels it.

The Muscles That Move Us

People tend to focus on shortening the muscle when they want to get stronger and tend to focus on stretching when they feel tight. However, it's not always that simple. You've probably had the thought, *my hamstrings are tight.* Feeling a sense of tightness in a muscle is a common complaint. It's normal. The gut reaction is to stretch. You may have thought of a particular muscle as tight, short, or strong, but it isn't quite so simple. Your hamstrings may feel tight because they are short and really strong, but they can also feel tight if they are weak. This is where a dialogue with your practitioner is key. The more information you provide them about what you are feeling, the better they should be able to guide you through a movement or help you decide if a movement is right for you.

There is a constant game of tug-of-war happening between all of our muscles every time we move. Muscles function by contracting. When one muscle shortens, the opposing muscle needs to lengthen. Even when a muscle is lengthening, it is contracting. This is an important concept. Eccentric muscle work (the kind that happens when a muscle gets longer) is essential, because it creates a strong, long body. Picture doing a bicep curl with a weight. When you bend the elbow, bringing the hand to your shoulder, that is *concentric* (shortening).

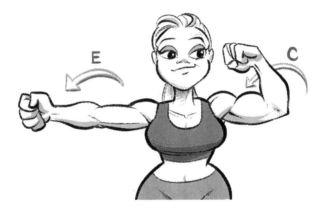

When you lengthen the arm and lower the weight, that's *eccentric* (lengthening). And when you pick a place and hold the weight there without moving, that is *isometric*. Our goal for the body should be to create two well-balanced tug of war teams, each side momentarily moving ahead and then behind throughout our whole day. We need the body to compete in the long game.

Eccentric contractions—the movements where the muscle gets long while it is loaded—are a dream come true. They are the balance between stretch and strength. When we control movement as we lengthen a muscle, we become stronger as we increase flexibility. As an added bonus, we all have more strength when we work muscles eccentrically. You may not be able to do a pull-up, but you might be able to start at the top of the pull-up bar and lower yourself down.

Ideally, all the muscles in our body are the winning combination of long and strong, that wondrous idealism eccentric contractions create. Work and stretch together: that is the dream team.

Movement Break: Tipping Bird

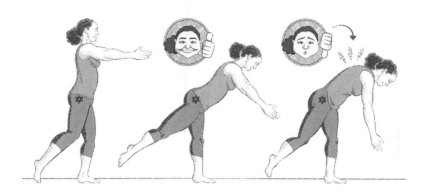

This movement will help you feel an eccentric contraction at work. It is especially beneficial for those of us who sit a lot. We tend to have short, tight hamstrings (back of the thigh), and we need to lengthen them in a functional way. Remember those toys shaped like a bird with a little water held in the bottom that can rock back and forth indefinitely? We are going to mimic the tipping bird with our own body to lengthen and strengthen our hamstring eccentrically. Try this:

- Put all your weight in one leg with a soft bend in the knee (not locked).

- Place the other leg slightly behind you so the toes are barely touching the floor. Hands can be on hips or reaching out in front, but either way they just go along for the ride.

- Stay tall and hinge forward at the hip of the floor leg (this might be a very small move) letting your trunk hinge forward as you lift your back leg. The torso and back leg should stay in-line with each other. Try not to round the back. Try to keep the hips squared off forward.

- Then hinge back to the start position.

- NOTE: Notice your sitz bone, the bony protrusion at the bottom of your butt. Keep pulling that bone up to the ceiling, and when it cannot go any farther, that is your end range-of-motion for now. When the hamstring and sitz bone cannot move any more, that is where you stop. Less is more.

- Repeat 10 times on each side.

- Tip: Losing your balance? Put a hand on the wall.

Let's return to the idea that if we feel tight, we need to stretch. I'm not trying to talk you out of stretching, but here is a new way to consider tight muscles: *tight equals strong and weak equals long couldn't be more wrong.* Part of a muscle can be tight. Part of that same muscle can be long and overly flexible. An individual muscle can have variability within it. So, if movements you have tried in the past have not gotten you the results you wanted, understanding what is causing the sensation of tightness provides more options to explore.

For simplicity, we are using words like "weak" or "strong," because those are the terms we can easily relate to as concepts. The problem is that we tend to think weak is bad and strong is good. Being weak (underdeveloped) or strong (overdeveloped) can both create problems. It is a matter of degree. One part is pulling more than the other, and what we are really searching for is balance between the two. Opposing muscles need to coexist constantly or else one "strong" muscle will require a "weak" muscle in order to function. Likewise, we can also be strong (a positive connotation) but not have functional strength. Perhaps we can lift a lot of weight at the gym, but if that does not translate into the chores or movement required in daily life, it may not be worth all the heavy lifting.

At first glance, this seems complicated, but, in fact, it provides possibilities. It now makes sense why you have never gained flexibility trying to stretch your hamstrings. You can stretch them day and night, but maybe you need to strengthen your quads (the opposing muscle) so that the two muscles are better balanced. Rarely will targeting one specific place resolve what hurts. Stretching a tight muscle will not work in isolation in the body. Our entire body is in a partnership and has to work together to promote change.

Types of Muscles

Our bodies consist of different types of muscles that perform different roles. We tend to care about our big, strong muscles, the ones we can see like our pecs, glutes, quads, and six-packs. Not that those muscles are not important. They are often big, major movers, known as *superficial muscles,* because they tend to be on top near the skin, close to the surface.

If we are going to use stereotypes to prove a point (and we are), our superficial muscles are like the high school jocks. They are big and tough and can take down another football player. They get us to the championship, because they are strong and can push us through a crisis and a challenge. But for all of their brute strength, they require rest, downtime, and recovery. They were not made to support our posture all day. They find the tedious work of holding us up draining and fatiguing. If we ask them to do the refined work of the smaller stabilizer muscles, they do the job with compression and tension, putting pressure on joints. These guys cannot be subtle.

Our *local stabilizer muscles* are the nerds in school, desperately scrambling to keep it all together. They are very bright and know what we need to stay balanced. They have analyzed the long game and understand what we need to win. When working properly, they provide our brain with a lot of sensory feedback about where we are in space. They are micromanagers who help with all the small movements that need to take place within our joint space to create the big moves the jocks like. They are anticipatory. They know the fate of the body first and try to adjust so that we remain structurally sound to all the pressure the superficial muscles and the world place on the body. But they are small, puny in comparison to the superficial jocks. And if one is going to overpower the other, the jocks will win and the stabilizers will shut down. Between these extremes is the teacher's pet. Known as *global stabilizers*, these muscles exist in both realms. They can be deep stabilizers or superficial muscles. They are pretty keen observers and help us decelerate our movement (eccentric contractions). They do it all.

We live in a world where we often get caught up thinking bigger is better. It is not necessarily so. Those big muscles we all want to look nice cannot do their jobs without the little guys. Getting to know some of your nerdy muscles is vital when you are in pain. They are your key to finding homeostasis in the body. But to balance something, we have to know it exists. Hence, we discuss some of the muscles and the following muscle haiku on the next few pages:

> Oh, my sweet muscles
> They call you superficial
> But how you move me

Some Muscles You Should Know About

There will not be a test after this section. These are some of the muscles I hope you grow to love and stop taking for granted. Understanding how they function (and that they exist) is key to helping you ease pain.

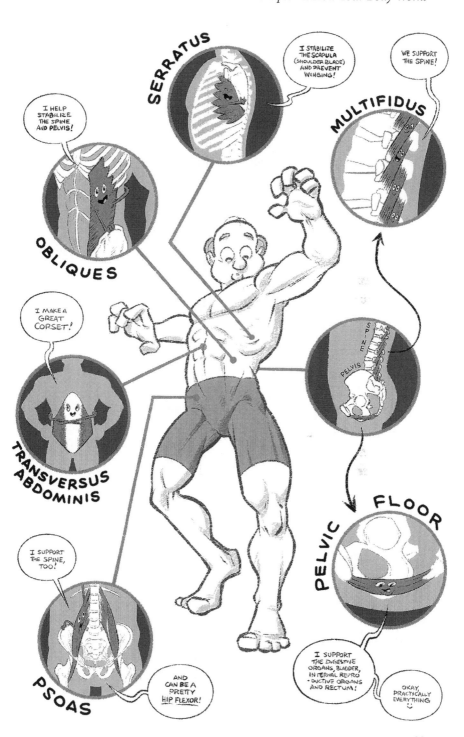

Local Stabilizers

Transversus Abdominis (TA): In my dreams, rather than drooling over pinups of six-pack abs, every man and woman swoons for an active, healthy TA. It is your deepest abdominal muscles, wrapping around you like a corset but not in a bad way. Since women destroyed and disfigured themselves for years by wearing corsets to create a particular physique, the corset has a bad rap and rightly so. But the TA is a supportive corset. It aids in spine stabilization. And learning to engage your TA is one of the best things you can do for back support to alleviate chronic back pain (see the Movement Break: TA Engagement on page 158).

Multifidus: These are multiple little guys running up your entire back between each vertebra. They help stabilize the spine.

Serratus Anterior: One of my favorites but also a problem child, the serratus is known as the boxing muscle, because it allows your scapula (shoulder blade) to protract (come forward around the body) as you would need it to when throwing a punch. The serratus is also partly responsible for keeping the scapula flat against the rib cage. This matters because your ribcage is vital to the mobility of your shoulder joint. When the scapula sticks out, it is called *winging* or an *anterior tip*. You can often see it on extremely slender super models. One part or the entire inside edge of their shoulder blade will pop up away from their ribs. That is not supposed to happen. That is a sign of an unhappy shoulder. If the shoulder blade does not rest on the ribs where it is supposed to, it might lead to pain, discomfort, and reduced range of motion. If shoulder pain nags you, you should get to know the serratus. It is also involved in breathing. Go, serratus. This muscle rocks!

Pelvic Floor Muscles (commonly known as Kegels): Many men do not realize they have Kegels, but both men and women have them. There are numerous reasons to appreciate your pelvic floor muscles. For women: when pelvic floor muscles are working right, they keep us from peeing every time we sneeze, and they hold all our internal organs inside of us. For men: pelvic floor muscles are vital for sustained and controlled erections. Are you more interested in your pelvic floor muscles yet?

!WARNING! Ranting diatribe to follow. The National Institutes of Health estimates that over a third of women have a pelvic floor disorder. This means that most women you meet pee a little when they sneeze, cough, laugh, run, or do a jumping jack. It is common, and there is no need for embarrassment. Who am I kidding? Pissing yourself is embarrassing, but at least you should not feel alone. Still, we should not accept this as normal. A few years ago, a CrossFit video went viral idolizing women peeing (more than a little) when they lifted heavy weight. It was a unifying video showing that this happens to the best of us, and that it is cool. I'm glad they wanted women to feel normal, but I'm not glad that they acted like this was okay. It is not okay. It is a sign something is wrong. If you pee when you do not want to, you have a degree of pelvic prolapse.

At its worst, pelvic prolapse can involve your bladder or uterus falling into or out of your vagina. This is NOT normal, though it is far too common. It should not and does not have to happen. In France after a woman has a baby, it is standard for her to go to physical therapy until her pelvic floor is back in tip-top shape. This protocol is not typical in the United States. We need to bring back healthy pelvic floors for women. Can you see the signage now?

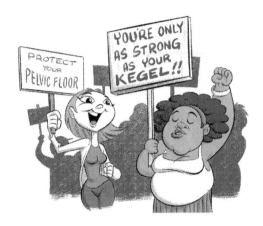

To find your pelvic floor, stop peeing midstream. What you feel when you stop midstream is engagement of the pelvic floor. That is a useful tool for finding your Kegels, but like every muscle, the pelvic floor is a bit more complicated. Not only is it difficult for some people, particularly for menopausal women, to engage their Kegels on command, but you also need to make sure you have some control over the whole muscle from front to back. (You are trying to do a Kegel now, aren't you?) While less common, problems can also develop if those muscles running between your pubic bone, tailbone, and sitz bones are overdeveloped. Like any muscle, whether over- or underdeveloped, a pelvic floor imbalance can cause a leaky bladder and result in low back pain. Yes, your pelvic floor and the state of your back are related.

The TA, the multifidus, and the pelvic floor muscles intuitively activate milliseconds before every movement, or at least they are supposed to. Without even noticing it, these three muscles automatically engage before every movement we make, even an unexpected sneeze. They trigger because they are stabilizers and aim to keep the spine safe. The little guys protect us with every move. If you pee a little when you sneeze, you feel firsthand that those muscles are not engaging properly. For many with chronic back pain, they do not engage at all. The multifidi actually atrophy, or waste away, and are replaced with fat. When we need them most, they aren't there to support us. If they're not working, we need to retrain them to work. Luckily, we can.

Global Stabilizers

Obliques

While we pine for six-pack abs, it is not the abdominal muscle that creates pain relief by stabilizing the spine and pelvis. For that, we can thank our obliques. These are the muscles that wrap around our waist. They allow us to twist, bend sideways, and round forward (flexion of the trunk). They are extremely versatile. These four muscles basically surround our abdomen, connecting our ribs and pelvis. They are global stabilizers, so they can act superficially but also play a role in stabilizing in a way the six-pack muscle cannot. Getting your obliques involved in ab exercises (like a basic crunch) instead of depending on your six-pack muscle works more and larger muscles while creating a strong support system for your back and pelvis. If you want pelvic stability, you want strong, functional obliques. As an added bonus, your internal obliques connect to the fascia in your lower back (thoracolumbar fascia), making them vital to lower back health. (Don't worry, there will be more on fascia, since it is likely key to your pain.)

Local and Global Stabilizers

Psoas

Ah, the supple psoas (pronounced: So-As). If you experience hip pain, you already may be familiar with this guy. It is known as the filet mignon of our muscles or the fight-or-flight muscle. We often call it a hip flexor, which means it allows us to lift or move our legs forward, but it is so much more.[30] It connects to all the vertebrae in our lumbar spine (low back) and is often the culprit contributing to hip pain and low back pain. It is there to help stabilize the spine. The psoas ends on one of two vertebrae. Which of the two vertebrae it settles on in any individual, we do not know, but the answer affects your flexibility. When you look at your neighbor in a fitness class and think they are more flexible than you are, remember, unlike Superman, none of us can see inside anyone else's body. Individuals will have a tendency toward increased flexibility based on where their psoas muscles connect. You cannot change that.

Fascia

I like talking about fascia a lot. I'm fascinated by the connective tissue running throughout our whole body. My mom once asked me, "Why should anyone care about fascia?" My jaw dropped. She got an earful. Please, let me share my love with you. I promise to keep it short with just the highlights.

Fascia is the connective tissue that runs along every surface of the body, intertwining itself with everything else. It encases the organs, muscles, bones, nerves, and other soft tissue, like a sausage casing or the sections of an orange where each large and tiny segment of juice is held together by a sleek, thin film. The muscles themselves are encased, but so is each muscle fiber. Fascia wraps around every fiber of your muscle individually like a sleeve; then a few fibers are held together by another sleeve, and a large bundle is held together within that sleeve, and on and on, with more wrapping around the whole bundle of fibers. Fascia abounds everywhere in our body.

---

30 The psoas has always been considered a hip flexor, but there is now some debate as to whether that is truly the role it plays. It may solely be engaging in hip flexion to stabilize the spine. It is possible it is not technically involved in the movement of hip flexion.

There are different types of fascia that serve different purposes. Fascia helps us move. It helps us recoil, use, and store force in movement. It lets our parts glide so that when we move our skin, tendons and muscles do not stick to our other parts. Each part can move smoothly alongside the other. Most people probably do not know fascia exists, yet without it all our parts would be stuck. Fascia basically acts like a lubricant between all our moving parts, causing trouble when it develops scars or adhesions. Fascia separates and defines different structures of the body, creating a buffer between them. It ensures our organs don't bang together when we jump. It joins structures together, as it does when it connects a muscle to a bone via a tendon. Fastened between all the structures of the body, fascia is much more than the packing material and glue it was assumed to be for years.

Fascia is the stuff in between all the other stuff. And somehow, though it is everywhere, for quite some time, we thought it did not do anything significant. We could not have been more wrong. Recently, it was "discovered" that a particular type of fascia is probably an organ. They have named it *interstitium* (pronounced: inter-stich-e-um). It is a continuous, fluid-filled space between the muscles, organs, and circulatory system. Scientists believe understanding this organ better may help them understand how cancer spreads. Perhaps, just like the way we draw blood now to learn about our health and diseases, we might be able to draw the interstitial fluid and learn about diseases faster. There is some very promising research in your fascia!

The fascia also plays an essential role in posture and organization of the body in movement. It is the organ of form. This all-encompassing collagen can help the muscles do their job. When healthy fascia remains springy (for lack of a better word) in movement, the muscles can use less energy and will not fatigue as quickly, because the fascia takes some of the burden of force and helps the body return to its "normal" shape. Fascia is your friend for all kinds of movement.

Without trying to get too scientific, our fascia is entwined with our extracellular matrix (ECM), all the stuff in our body that is not living cells that our living cells are hanging onto. What is exciting about ECM is that it appears to play a huge role in regeneration of wounds, injuries, and tissues, like muscles. ECM with physical therapy was utilized in five cases to help initiate regrowth in muscles of veterans and civilians who had lost between 60 to 90 percent of a muscle.[31] As we learn more, this is an area rife with potential to help us heal in endless ways.

Movement Break: Feel Your Fascia

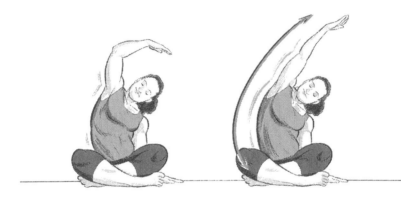

You can feel your fascia. It is believed we have six times more sensory nerve endings in fascia than in muscles, so your fascia provides your brain with a lot of feedback. To feel your fascia, play with different stretches.

---

31 NBC News, "Experimental Treatment Regrows Muscle in Injured Men's Legs," April 30, 2014, www.nbcnews.com/health/health-news/experimental-treatment-regrows-muscle-injured-mens-legs-n94101.

The Back Line

- Lie down on your back.

- Straighten one leg up to the ceiling like you are going to do a hamstring stretch. Hold the leg with your hands if that adds comfort.

- Flex the foot of the leg in the air by pulling the toes toward the nose. Try to lengthen out your heel.

- Feel the heaviness in the glute and pelvis.

- Think of lengthening out the crown of your head.

- Notice the difference between flexing the foot and letting it relax.

- Notice the difference between lengthening out the spine as you hold the stretch. As the stretch spreads throughout the back of your leg and maybe even to your back, you can feel a long line of pull, not simply one muscle. It sometimes feels more like the skin is getting taut. When you can feel a long line of one stretch passing joints, you are feeling your fascia.

- Repeat on the other side.

The Side Line

- Sit on the floor with legs crossed lotus style, if that is comfortable.

- Bend to one side, placing that hand on the floor to help support you and the other arm over your head like you are a ballerina.

- Take a deep breath and then sit back up.

- Return to the same stretch, but this time straighten the arm over your head as if you are actively reaching for where the wall and ceiling meet.

- Notice how the stretch feels differently when all you did was reach out your arm.

- Repeat on the other side.

Play with it. If you don't know what you are feeling right away or don't feel anything, don't worry. It might take some experimentation.

Bones

We have 206 bones in our bodies, a quarter of which comprise our feet. From the feet up, bones stack above each other to create our posture. They could not do it alone. It would be impossible to stack all our bones up on top of each other without our muscles and tendons to hold them together. We would have a pile of bones. They are structured to work in conjunction with everything else (fascia, muscles, tendons, ligaments) to have an upright posture. Picture a dinosaur exhibit except with human bones showing human structure. We have a very large skull that sits on top of a little cervical (neck) spine. We have a spine with curvature that enables upright posture. In addition to providing our basic shape and structure, bones are protective like a turtle shell: the ribs protect our lungs and heart, and our skull protects our brain.

Our bones are designed to be light and strong in order to make movement easy. When compared by weight, bones can take five times more load than steel. They are also more elastic, which means they have some give and pliability. If they were as heavy as steel, we would not be able to hold ourselves up or walk. Making up about a sixth of our body weight, our lightweight bones were made for walking, movement, and pliability. Our muscles attach to our bones via tendons, and together they make us move.

As we come to understand that all of our parts work together, it is important to note that movement is essential for bone health. Both aerobic and strength training have been shown to increase bone density, which is especially important for us as we age, and particularly important for women or anyone with osteoporosis or osteopenia. A dozen studies have shown the significant effects of strength training on bone density, making that the go-to movement for bone health.[32] A 2000 study looked at aging adults to compare whether using machines with lighter weight and more repetitions (what they termed "moderate intensity weight lifting") or using free weights with heavier weight and fewer repetitions ("high intensity weight lifting") yielded better results.[33] Both were good, but the free weights had slightly higher results.

The science shows any activity is good for our health. When we are physically active, it puts a healthy stress on our bones that encourages the growth of *osteoblasts*, the cells that help us build bone. In addition to protecting our innards and giving our muscles something to move, the bones produce red blood cells to carry oxygen throughout our body and fuel our muscles and white blood cells for our immune system. Bones are alive. They repair themselves. As with every system in the body, moving helps them do their job.

32 Jennifer E. Layne and Miriam E. Nelson, "The Effects of Progressive Resistance Training on Bone Density: A Review," *Medicine & Science in Sports and Exercise* 31, no. 1 (Jan 1999): 25–30, https://doi.org/10.1097/00005768-199901000-00006.
33 Heidi M. Weingart and Len Kravitz, "Resistance Training and Bone Mass," The University of New Mexico, 2001, https://www.unm.edu/~lkravitz/Article%20folder/bonemass.html.

Tendons and Ligaments

Tendons and ligaments are part of our connective tissue system. They are thick and almost ropey, made primarily of collagen and a little elastin, and are generally durable. You may be able to picture a white tendon connecting a muscle to the bone the way your typical anatomy book would draw them, but in reality, the ends of the tendons blend into the muscle, becoming the fascia that wraps around and through every muscle fiber like the thin film around each orange segment. Tendons attach muscles to bones. Ligaments attach bones to bones. So your Achilles' tendon connects your calf muscles to the heel bone (calcaneus), and the ACL (anterior cruciate ligament) in the knee connects two bones, the shinbone (tibia) and thighbone (femur). These structures in the body are part of our web that holds us together. They are all interconnected.

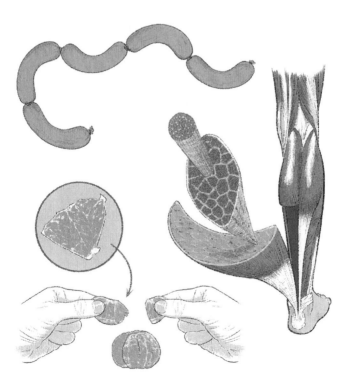

Tendons and ligaments may take a long time to heal, but they do heal with time, although the best course of action to assist healing is still up for debate. Every person and every tendon is different, but in the case of tendinopathy, strength training of the tendon and muscle is required. This represents a shift in approach, since advice in the past has typically emphasized the importance of rest and ice. If those tools help, you can use them, but continuing a strength program geared toward you and your specific injury is more likely to reduce pain and restore function.[34] The proper course of action could differ based on the individual, which tendon in the body is injured, and which part of a specific tendon is injured.

Muscles and tendons work together, so if a tendon is injured, the local muscle can sometimes do additional work to support it. If a muscle is very tight, the tendon can stretch a bit to compensate. That is why it is important to be gentle on your body when you stretch. If the muscle cannot handle the stretch and you overstretch it, the tendon will take up the slack. Once your tendons are slack, it is much harder to restrengthen them. Think of an overly stretched elastic band. Muscles have a lot more give-and-take than tendons.

In addition to bones, tendons, ligaments, fascia, and muscle, you also have nerves, a circulatory system, organs, and hormones in your body. All the intertwined parts matter for your health and wellness and living a life without pain. Our anatomy lesson covered the areas that are often related to musculoskeletal pain. We will touch on the nervous system in the next chapter because it is the nervous system's role in pain that may be a part of society's pain problem.

---

34 Karen Litzy, "201: Busting Tendinopathy Myths with Dr. Jill Cook" *Healthy, Wealthy, Smart Podcast*, February 29, 2016.

CHAPTER 5: HOW YOUR BODY PARTS INTEGRATE AND WORK TOGETHER

Now that we know the basic parts, we need to understand how they work together. We are about to dive a little deeper and explain our relationship to them and how they are supposed to work in a combined and real way. Why does this information matter? In part, we have misconceptions about movement, pain, and why we hurt. If you learn newer concepts, a world of possibility will open up to help you keep moving. This information can rebuild hope where it is currently lost, creating potential and possibility. Especially if you are someone who feels movement hasn't helped in the past, having more information and understanding will create more options that I hope encourage you to experiment and try moving again.

For the health of our bodies and brains, we have to move. But we need to move from the proper place to create worthwhile, potentially permanent changes. Pain is a pattern. In order to unwind a pattern, you have to go inside your own body, pay attention, retrain muscles and nerves, and create new configurations of movement to figure out how to move effortlessly and set that movement as your new default. Once you're out of pain, the movement should naturally require less intentional concentration. It's time to reconsider movement in your body.

The Brain/Body Connection

The brain has good intentions, but sometimes it can get the wrong signal. The pain loop, where the brain gets wired to believe we are in pain, may be part of the chronic pain syndrome plaguing our society. If your brain thinks you are in pain, you are in pain. For example, if you see you have a bulging disc and you are experiencing pain, you might be afraid to move in certain ways. According to Dr. Adriaan Louw, physical therapist and co-founder of the International Spine and Pain Institute, when people are informed that 40 percent of people with bulging discs don't feel pain, they feel more comfortable trying to move.[35] Some physical issues do not guarantee pain even though we associate them with pain. This does not mean you should not be attentive to your pain. Part of what we do not yet fully understand is why some people have pain when others do not. A number of complicated issues are involved in the pain loop, but simply knowing pain is not a guarantee has helped people find relief. The fact that you are in pain now does not mean you will be in pain tomorrow or a year from now.

One theory on some types of chronic pain proposes that our nervous system crossed its wires. The brain might get so used

---

35 Adriaan Louw et al., "The Clinical Application of Teaching People About Pain," *Physiotherapy Theory and Practice* 32, no. 5 (2016): 385–95, https://doi.org/10.1080 /09593985.2016.1194652.

to signaling pain that even when the tissue is no longer in pain, the brain continues to tell us we are. The nerves have become oversensitized and want to keep us from getting reinjured even if we are completely safe. We need to consider teaching ourselves the old Apple motto: Think Different.

While our brain signals our body to move for basic activity, we don't actually have to think about it once we know how to do it. If you had to consider everything that was going on in your body each time you walked, you could not maintain a simple conversation about the weather and walk at the same time. This is where we have some degree of muscle memory. Once we have established a pattern, our body can just do it, Nike style. When you laugh about not being able to rub your belly and pat your head at the same time, realize that your body is doing far more complicated movements all the time, practically every second you are in motion. We take them all for granted because they have become easy and commonplace for us. Learning something new feels tough. With persistence, one day that challenging move might take no thought at all. One day, something that causes pain may no longer hurt. Certain movements—good and bad, pain-relieving and pain-inducing—become a memorized routine.

Once a pianist conquers a complicated piece, the speed at which her fingers tickle the ivories is too fast to have signals firing back and forth from the fingers to the brain. After years of experience and repetition, not every movement has to pass through the brain for approval. We just go. Our brains don't think about every individual action required to walk. We just walk. We thought about it as toddlers, but now we walk mindlessly. Just as the complicated activities we utilize daily, like walking or typing on a keyboard, can be done without conscious thought, pain, too, can be a signal that gets wired without the brain's approval. Sometimes a pain signal gets stopped by cells in the spinal column that don't allow the brain to review them. That's one way we get stuck in an endless cycle of pain.

> *Automaticity: the ability to do things without occupying the mind with the low-level details required, allowing it to become an automatic response pattern or habit. It is usually the result of learning, repetition, and practice.*

The brain and nervous system are *neuroplastic*, which means they can learn and change. While we don't fully understand where and how we can change in every situation, this is an area of great potential for rewiring and reducing pain. That pianist who plays fast sequences has less brain activity than a non-piano player when attempting any task that involves both hands. The brain has already learned how to do complicated tasks with both hands. The wiring is set. Now she can do it, even if there is no piano involved. Her experience automatically makes her hands better at two-handed complicated tasks.

The ability to "just do it" is what makes one athlete or pianist better than the next, according to research led by Eitan Globerson and Israel Nelken in Jerusalem.[36] When we transfer what we understand about piano players to athletes performing fast, complicated tasks, the better the athlete is at not thinking about the task; letting her body "just do it" translates to better performance, even if she is less physically fit than her competitor who is stuck in her own head. Once you know it, you know it forever. Thinking can hinder you. However, if you know it's wrong (e.g., a chronic pain condition), thinking is the piece of the puzzle that will correct the faulty pattern. You can reprogram your movement patterns.

---

36 Eitan Globerson and Israel Nelken, "The Neuro-Pianist," *Frontiers in Systems Neuroscience* 7 (Jul 2013), https://doi.org/10.3389/fnsys.2013.00035.

Feeling Is the Art of Healthy Moving

When I was training to become a Pilates instructor, we did an exercise to help us learn gentle tactile cueing during exercises. We placed a piece of hair under a thin phone book page (harder to come by these days) and then ran our fingers across the page with our eyes closed until we sensed the hair. Once found, we turned a second page over the hair and again searched for the fine tresses now hidden by two phone book pages with our fingertip. How many pages could we add and still find the hair? It was a struggle for me. Though I have trained myself to feel more, I have never been good at noticing gentle sensations in my body. I prefer firm massages or foam rollers over a gentle relaxing massage.

When I used to work for the Mark Twain House & Museum in Hartford, Connecticut, occasionally a blind student would be on a group tour. Since the child couldn't see the objects in the house, after the tour we'd provide a box of fabrics and materials that were similar to objects in the home for the student to touch. One day, I was taking a young girl through the box after her house tour and handed her a black lace cloth. She felt it and said, "Oh, what beautiful butterflies." I smiled, thinking how sweet it was that she pretended she could see patterns in the fabric. I'd done this program a few times, so I knew what everything looked like. When the girl left, I started putting everything away. As I picked up the black lace, I noticed it had a pattern of beautiful butterflies that I had never seen. I stood in awe for a moment. A young child without sight had shown me a part of the world I'd missed. Where my sense of sight was lacking, her sense of touch was profound. Touch is vital to life.

What we feel when we move is important. An ability to feel subtle movement or subtle engagement of a particular muscle can help us unwind pain. If we are unable to make big moves for a while during a recovery phase, being able to sense and make small adjustments can help us develop bigger and bigger moves over time. Also, learning what you feel in your body helps you react as needed or provide feedback to a practitioner who is guiding you. If a certain exercise is intended for you to feel it in your glutes but you feel it in your back, that feeling can be the beginning of learning to activate muscles in a different way so the back doesn't overwork and the intended muscle starts to fire. As you understand what you feel in your body more, you will gain confidence differentiating between acceptable amounts of pain for you, and what you want and should call "uncle" on. If you are not paying attention to what you feel in your body when moving, you will miss opportunities for beneficial change, much like I'd been missing the butterflies in the fabric.

Is Your Body Flexible or Tight?

We tend to admire flexibility; practically everyone I meet craves it. Flexibility is important. The simple sit-rise test proves that both strength and flexibility are required for longevity. Brazilian physician Claudio Gil Araujo developed the sit-rise test. His team rated over 2,000 participants in a study looking to see how easily the participants could get from a standing position to a seated position and back up again without the use of hands or any assistance. Dr. Araujo designed the study when he realized some of his older patients who excelled at aerobic exercises like running and biking died earlier than their health testing would indicate. He wondered why they were dying if they appeared to have healthy hearts and lungs and deduced that something else needed consideration when measuring factors that influence lifespan. The key might be anaerobic activity (movement that doesn't require oxygen or improve cardiovascular capacity). To function optimally, the body requires strength and flexibility. The proper combination of both enables us to balance without falling over, and get up and down off the floor with ease.

Movement Break: Sit-Rise Test

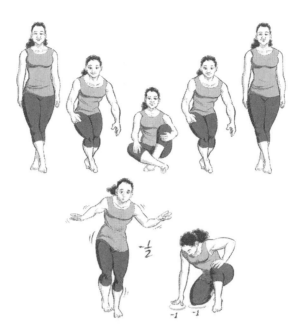

Here's how the sit-rise test works. You start with 10 points. You can lose up to five on the way down and five on the way back up. (If you have hip or knee replacements, do NOT try this test. You are exempt.)

1) Take off your shoes.

2) Start standing, legs crossed one foot in front of the other.

3) Lower your butt down onto the floor with control. Deduct a point for each hand or knee that touches the floor or a piece of furniture on the way down. If you wobble or lose your balance at any time, deduct half a point. However, use your body or a chair for assistance if you currently need it. It's not worth falling over to complete this test.

4) From the seated position with legs crossed, tailor, pretzel, or lotus style, try to stand back up without using your hands or flinging yourself forward. Again, deduct a point for each hand or knee that touches the floor or a piece of furniture on the way up. Wobbling costs half a point.

NOTE: Some people find this easier to do if they reverse the crossed leg position, letting their feet go out wide and their knees buckle in, known as the "W-Sit."

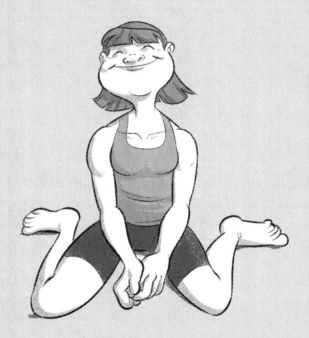

While you may see little kids choose the W-Sit position, if this is your happier place as an adult, it's unlikely your knees are happy or will have a lifelong happiness. If you notice this tendency in your body, for the future longevity of your knees and hips, consider exercises in the hip section of this book that focus on lateral rotation and outer thigh strength.

Your ability to complete this test is linked to your longevity. If you score three points or fewer, your chance of dying in the next five years is five times greater. Every point you earn represents a 20 percent decrease in mortality from all causes. If you scored an eight, feel great. Does your score scare you? Or were you pleasantly surprised by your results? If you scored under three, don't panic. It is not a death sentence. You can increase your flexibility and strength, and are in control of a lot of what happens in and to your body. Remember, the score is an indicator of probability, not a guarantee of fate. We all beat the odds. My grandfather lived for 90 years, even though his mom was told he wouldn't survive infancy. After contracting rheumatic fever as a child, he was told he wouldn't live past thirteen. He fought in WWII and survived to tell the stories to his grandchildren. Don't get down. Get motivated to change your patterns and behavior.

The real message is that we need to be *flexible enough*. Your body doesn't demand the suppleness of a ballerina. The graceful moves of a dancer are beautiful and impressive, but if you're not a ballerina, it's okay. Besides, ballerinas often pay the price for extreme flexibility at some point. Athletes, gymnasts, and dancers often develop pain and injuries later in life. The extremely physically fit are not exempt from pain. They used their body in ways that often pushed it beyond normal limits. A baseball pitcher may have multiple shoulder surgeries. What they do is spectacular. We admire it. But it is hard on the body. People who can sit down, spread their legs, fold forward, and touch their chest to the floor are *hypermobile*. If you can pull your thumb back to your wrist, it's a neat party trick, but your joint wasn't intended to have that much range of motion. Hypermobility is more common in women, and it may lead to pain for a variety of reasons. Hypermobile people often feel the sensation that they are tight and hanker for a stretch but find no relief from it. Very often, they overstretch, exacerbating the problem. Hypermobility causes joint instability, because the tendons and ligaments tend to be slack. Generalized, chronic pain is common for hypermobile people. This, in fact, might be a part of the puzzle for you.

When your tendons and ligaments are loose, your muscles have to take up the burden. Hypermobile people greatly benefit from body weight and strength training exercises because their muscles need to be stronger to pick up the workload for the tendons that are slacking off. But movement for the hypermobile can often be painful. Start slowly and ease into the movement. We are all individuals. Some of us are born more flexible than others. Some have a tendency to be stronger or faster. We often push ourselves past our personal normal, but eventually something else will give. Often what suffers are tendons and ligaments. Some people are born with loose tendons and ligaments; some people create them by overstretching. At times, our tendon length and flexibility is determined by our hormones. Pregnant women have a hormone called *relaxin* that creates looser, more flexible joints so the pelvis can expand during childbirth, but during this time all their joints are looser.

Are you starting to see how pain and movement is more complicated than we first thought? Notice changes in your body. If you have lost flexibility or suddenly feel tight, that's important, because it is a change in your normal. Otherwise, let's be happy with being flexible enough. Ask yourself: Why am I stretching? What's my goal? If it is flexibility for flexibility's sake, that's not a great motivator or even a really good reason. If you have decided to take up ice-skating and there is a new move you are working on, that would make sense. (Are you scoffing at adult-onset-desire-to-skate? It's real. And I know people—okay, a person—who came down with it.) Maybe you have noticed a loss in flexibility, and you are concerned and want to maintain the flexibility you have. That's a fantastic reason to stretch. It is likely, though, that you will achieve your goal faster if you incorporate more movement throughout the day.

If you think you are tight and inflexible, try the sit-rise test. It's a better indicator of the balance between our strength and flexibility. (I wish our schools would include this as part of physical education, since it's such an important movement.) If you can't do the sit-rise test yet, try building up to it with a few of these tips.

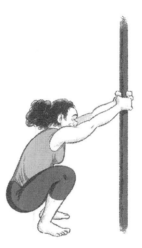

- Do deep and regular squats. You may need to hang onto a supportive structure at first in order to sit back into the squat. I use the edge of my kitchen sink, but make sure whatever you use can support your body weight. Hang onto the sink (or a safe object) and get used to existing in that position. NOTE: the deep squat is not for everyone. The way our bones fit together, the length of our legs, and the flexibility of our ankles can make this move easier for some and nearly impossible for others. So try not to force yourself into a position the body isn't ready for. Regular squats are good too. Also, you can try sitting on a low object, like an ottoman or step stool. Keep finding lower objects as you get more comfortable. You'll notice in the picture that my pelvis is not in neutral. We are striving for a neutral pelvis in this position. I struggle with that, but still find the position very comfortable in my body.

- Try lying on your back. Pull one or both legs into your chest. Hold for 30 seconds at a time.

- Try sitting cross-legged (lotus style). If this position feels uncomfortable or unnatural, sit propped up on something higher. Gradually lower your sitting platform. If you start from a position of pain and discomfort, the body will never welcome you going there. Why would it? We are intelligent beings. And how can we unwind pain if the body learns that we constantly force it to be in pain when we move?

- Experiment with putting your socks on while balancing on one foot. When you do this, keep the knee of the leg that is lifted in toward your chest, not allowing the knee to splay out toward your shoulder. If this one doesn't work for you right away, lie down on your back to put your socks on and try to assume the same position without making balance part of the equation.

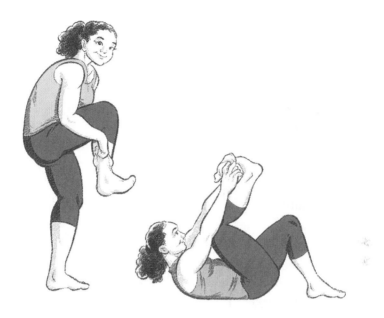

Turn these movements into daily tasks, like taking your vitamins. Pick one or three a day and spend up to five minutes working on improving your strength and flexibility, and ultimately improving your chance for healthy longevity. Five minutes a day can make a difference. Something is always better than nothing.

You've Lost That Spring in Your Step

For our overall well-being, it's important that we walk with a light, airy bounce in our step. If we walk or move with a pounding thud onto the floor, each step reverberates throughout our body, shocking and jarring the whole system. If walking feels laborious, you might be landing with a heavy stomp and then dragging your leg up like you are pulling it out of a mud pit. You might be walking like that and not even realize it, because it has become so normal to you. That's exhausting and is hard on the muscles and the joints. *Ouch, ouch, ouch*…that's every cell in your body reacting to how you've lost your springiness. If you are doing any movement and it starts to feel laborious, joints or ligaments start taking on the burden the muscles are meant to carry, which puts you at greater risk for injury.

Try to get a lighter spring in your step by thinking like a ninja during movement, whether in an exercise class or walking down the aisle at the grocery store. The ninja principle requires noticing that your movement is quiet and light, not hard and pounding. Consider concentrating on pushing off from your back leg and gliding forward almost like a speed skater with each step as you walk. Take smaller steps or bigger steps to see which makes you lighter on your feet or reduces pain in the body. When you go up and down stairs, how quiet can you be? Play with staying quiet at different paces and during different activities. You can move like a ninja at any fitness level.

You can also do bigger, sweeping fascial movements in the privacy of your own home. Gil Hedley is a self-taught anatomist with a PhD in ethics. In a lecture I attended, he talked about how he would do tai chi on the lakefront in Chicago during college. People would come up to him and tell him he had no chi. (Who has the gall to tell another person they have no chi?) Years later, he came to the conclusion that they had been right; he had no chi in his youth. Now, having studied fascia, he showed us how he moves: arms waving, body undulating, torso rippling. After the talk, I asked him what people say now when he moves like that. He said, "Oh, I don't do that in public." I laughed and understood why he felt that way. We are very judgmental about movement and tend to judge ourselves as much as we judge others. That judgement inhibits us, and our body suffers for it.

We need to try to get past our discomfort with moves that seem odd or silly. Fascia's fluid and elastic properties are meant to allow for more ease in movement so no piece of the puzzle falls to one small muscle. Movement involves the whole body with the muscles, tendons, and fascia operating together. For example, when you walk, your arms should swing. Tuck them into your pockets, cross your arms, or hold the phone up to your ear with one hand and that part of the movement disappears. Walking is a full-body workout and should involve your butt, abs, and back. And there should be buoyancy in each step. If you don't take advantage of your elasticity, then every movement is harder.

As elastic beings, we have to consider whole body movements with bends, spirals, and waves. That way a broader area can take on what could be seen as the burden for a small part of us and turn once-painful movement into a joy. Think of a baseball batter or a golfer winding up. They use their entire body, not only their arms, to hit the ball. They are capitalizing on stored elasticity. A baseball pitcher doesn't bring his pitching hand to his shoulder and toss the ball over the plate. He winds up with his whole body. The golfer doesn't tap the ball. She twists her entire body back before swinging. We intuitively know to recoil and release, and there are particular activities we instinctively wind up for. But if we aren't a golfer or our chances of playing for the Red Sox are over, we don't use these full ranges of motion—or windup methods—very often throughout our day or in life. Making time for full-body movement is beneficial to a functional system.

All this information may seem complicated, but it's important to expand our thinking beyond the two-dimensional framework we're accustomed to. If we think of ourselves as elastic, tensile beings with a connectedness among all our parts, rather than just one part being tight or strong, we can start to move in a way that enhances our whole body. This line of thinking creates more opportunity for change. The body has an amazing capacity for comfortable movement; we just need to remember how. Perhaps we have simply forgotten how to move with ease. We need to find our buoyancy, and that comes from understanding how we really move, how much support we have, and how we need to care for the different parts so they can work maximally using minimal effort. Learning to move better is actually the lazy man's dream. If you've had success getting out of pain with the tools you've always had, that's fantastic. If you haven't had success yet, it's time to add more tools to your movement and healthcare tool belt.

If you are jumping, walking, running, or doing any type of movement and it feels hard or strained, you're not capitalizing on the elasticity—the tensional springiness—of your own body. So how do you do that? Practice full-body, functional movement. Rethink what you are doing at the gym or on a walk. Try incorporating some windup movements (only if they don't hurt). Here are a few examples. They may feel funny, different, or uncomfortable at first, but stick with it.

Movement Break: Full-Body Soccer Kicks

Remember, if these moves hurt, skip them for now or work through whatever range is pain-free.

The Soccer Kick

- Stand next to a wall.

- Put one hand on the wall for balance and support.

- Shift your weight slightly into one foot so that you have room to swing the leg farthest from the wall.

- Bring the arm away from the wall overhead as far back as you comfortably can and your leg away from the wall as far behind you as it will travel comfortably, then let them swing forward as if their own weight and moment is carrying them.

- Repeat a few times until you feel loose.

- Repeat on other side.

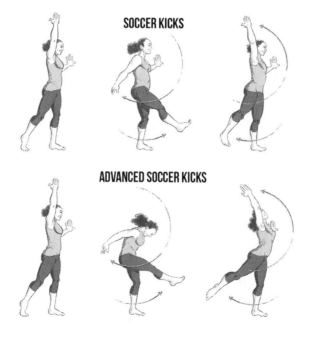

SOCCER KICKS

ADVANCED SOCCER KICKS

Advanced Soccer Kick

- Follow the same steps above with a couple of modifications.

- When you pull the limbs back, allow your chest to lift, bringing you into a slight backbend. Emphasize the bend up the upper back more than the lower back.

- As the limbs come forward, let your torso, head, and body round forward creating a fuller body movement.

Spinning Drum

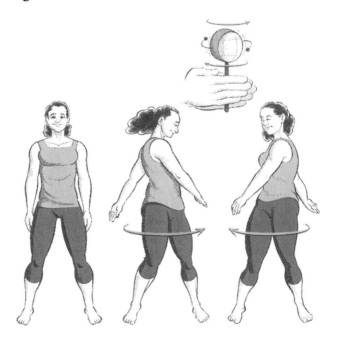

Remember when you were a kid and you had that hand-held drum with two beads attached to two strings? You turned it between your fingers and the beads flew through the air and beat the opposite sides of the drum. Picture that.

- Stand with feet shoulder-width apart

- Turn your torso from side to side and let your arms go along for the ride.

- Sometimes, keep your pelvis still only twisting from the waist up. Other times, allow the pelvis to move with you. Compare how stabilizing the pelvis or letting it move freely feels.

Get Creative

When it comes to movement, we always seem to be following the rules. This is proper swimming form. That is how we do the tango. As adults, we rarely make time for play, and our movements always seem prescribed. We put limits on our movement and stuff ourselves into a figurative box. We are afraid and embarrassed to move freely. But playful exploration can be helpful. Start moving and see what you like and what you are drawn to. You may discover that your body intrinsically knows what it needs if you provide it time to play and explore. The entire purpose is to move in ways that feel pleasurable. There is no judgement. If you need a little help getting started, try the Zeppelin in the Neck & Shoulder section or visualize your cat or dog stretching and mimic some of those moves. In Dick Van Dyke's book *Keep Moving: And Other Tips and Truths About Living Well Longer,* he recommends dancing everywhere. If you hear a good song, even as you are strolling down the grocery store aisle, he encourages you to start jiving to the beat. It's a great tip, though I think Dick Van Dyke can get away with it more easily than you or I can.

How We Feel

Everything we feel throughout the day is transmitted through our nervous system. It is a massive system. An adult has over 45 miles of nerves running like highways, carrying signals throughout the body. We have a central nervous system (the nerves in the brain and spinal column) and a peripheral nervous system (all the other nerves in the body). Both have voluntary and involuntary components. The *autonomic* is voluntary and vital; it manages the workings of all our organs. We do not have to tell our heart to beat because the autonomic nervous system just does it. And while we can control our breathing when we want to, breathing happens naturally, as does digestion.

The involuntary systems include: sympathetic, parasympathetic, and enteric (which controls the bowels). The *sympathetic* ("fight-or-flight") nervous system prepares us for action. If we need to run away from a bear or stay up all night to get an important presentation ready, the sympathetic system keeps us going. It directly links to stress, typically immediate stressors. The *parasympathetic* ("rest-and-digest") system allows us to relax, unwind, and let go. If you are in chronic pain, you need the parasympathetic system to encourage you to slow down, but often the body will stay tense as a protective mechanism, resulting in more or lingering pain. Our bodies remember experiences and can hold a grudge. Sometimes, we need to let go and break a cyclical pain pattern. To reduce pain, look for patterns you can reverse. Stop and ask, when did the pain really start? What moves still aggravate it, and is there any way I can alter those movements so they don't hurt or hurt less? What position can I get in that alleviates pain? It is the stopping, slowing down, becoming aware, and listening to your body throughout the day that will guide you out of pain.

The ability to feel is vital to living a quality life. When living with pain, it's easy to resent it, but shutting down our senses is not beneficial. Instead, we need to figure out what our sensations are trying to communicate to us. Most people don't enjoy pain and would happily give it up, but it is the body's coping mechanism. Next time something hurts and you are wishing you did not feel pain, realize that most people who have no sense of pain die prematurely. Without an ability to feel pain, we would often be injured by our own world, drinking something that scalds the esophagus, burning our retinas after looking at the sun, or losing toes to frost bite. A degree of pain keeps us alive by preventing us from engaging in activities that put our body in harm's way. That's where exteroception, proprioception, and interoception— the modes in which we perceive and feel sensations—become relevant.

The Feelings That Make Us Aware

When we feel the warm rays of the sun on our skin, pull our hand quickly away from the hot stove, or feel soothed by aloe vera, we are experiencing the sense of touch that we are most familiar with: *exteroception*. We see, hear, smell, and take in all sorts of sensation from the outside world. Our brain processes it, and we respond to the feedback from our surroundings. Basically, exteroception is what we feel externally. *Proprioception* is how we move and sense ourselves in space based on feedback from muscles, tendons, and joints. It is our sense of agility, balance, and coordination. Your ability to type on a computer or play the piano without looking at your fingers is due to proprioception. You have an idea of where all your parts exist in space without needing to see or hear them move. When sober, you can touch your fingers to your nose with your eyes closed. But when inebriated, your proprioceptive skills diminish. Suddenly, you can't pass a very basic sobriety test.

Interoception is our inner sensation stimulated by our organs. Hunger, thirst, arousal, feeling sick, an irritating itch, and the urge to use the bathroom all develop from signals inside our body, much of which is related to our autonomic nervous system (it happens without much thought from us). They are the sensations that are believed to provide our sense of self and our emotional awareness, and may explain our feeling of sentience, or what we as humans like to believe divides us from other animals.

Our nervous system is constantly providing sensation, internal and external, good and bad. Every moment it is trying to determine where we are in space and how to create equilibrium. Our body keeps our heart pumping, digests our food while not falling over, and maintains a temperature of 98.6°F no matter what happens around us. To accomplish this, our nervous system picks up on sensations we tend not to notice. To function in the world, we cannot notice everything we feel, but observing early signs is imperative to stopping pain before it starts and reducing pain quickly. More often than not, before we experienced pain, our body gave us warning signals that we ignored. Maybe we were young, busy, didn't pay attention, or didn't know it wasn't supposed to feel that way.

In Pilates, we often ask, "where do you feel this?" In my own practice, I have not always been able to acknowledge where or what I'm feeling, so I understand when my clients do not have an answer. I require a lot of sensation to provide feedback. I've learned to feel more, and that plays a huge role in my stopping pain before it starts. Just as we all have different hair color, leg length, and innate flexibility, our nervous systems operate differently. It is okay to feel what you feel, how you feel it. We all experience pain differently with different thresholds, yet we often try to compare pain. Are kidney stones as excruciating as giving birth? How did someone else react to a bee or jellyfish sting? How our pain compares to someone else's is irrelevant. We feel what we feel. I recommend scoring your pain by asking yourself on a scale of one to ten where your pain falls. It doesn't matter if someone else feels a five when you feel a seven. If that person stepped inside your body and had your nervous system, she would feel a seven, too. That number will provide feedback to you and your practitioner.

When you are frustrated by pain, remember it is our ability to feel our world that keeps us alive and functioning. Chronic pain is a terrible burden, but living with pain is better than living without the ability to feel sensation, and there are tools to reduce discomfort.

Pay Attention

We often ignore or miss sensations our body collects from the environment. Sometimes disregarding sensation is as vital as feeling it. The world would be too intense if we picked up on everything and reflected on it. Though not a current medical diagnosis, Sensory Processing Disorder seems to affect many children with autism and people with anxiety.[37] Loud noises, textures, or the pelting of the water during a shower can overwhelm people. They are processing sensation too much. The brain can be inundated by all the information it processes, or it can help us look past it. For example, the brain has structured your view so that you don't see your nose all the time, disrupting every gorgeous sunset. (You can see your nose now, can't you? Sorry. It will fade away again soon.)

We are not intended to notice how every part of us feels in every situation, but we also live in a hectic, crazed world where we are

---

37 Smitha Bhandari, editor, "Sensory Processing Disorder," *WebMD*, updated January 8, 2017, https://www.webmd.com/children/sensory-processing-disorder#2.

distracted and operating at an atypically fast pace. Throughout our day, it is very easy to miss or ignore what our body is telling us in order to complete necessary tasks. However, we don't want to miss important signals. Learning to listen to the signals the body provides is our first step in healing and reducing pain. If we do not listen, we wind up stuck in the pain loop, unsure of what is causing our pain, where it originates, or what moves feel good and safe.

Upon turning 25, I experienced a quarter-life crisis and decided that I needed to run a marathon now or never. Over a year earlier, I'd accepted my first full-time job and enrolled in graduate school, so time became limited (one of the best excuses for not exercising). My running and exercise routine ceased completely. Then one day, panicked by my race against time, I ran six miles. That convinced me to register for the Hartford Marathon. If I could run six miles, I falsely reasoned, then I could run 26.2. I completed two other six-mile runs before the big day. That was the extent of my training.

Looking back on that day through rose-colored glasses, I'd say it was mostly torture. It was pouring rain. Dead, trampled frogs littered the road. My shoes were sopping wet. To boost my ego, a couple who was walking the race overtook me, forcing me to recognize my running pace had deteriorated to less than a walking pace. Runners in Hartford have six hours to complete the course. With less than seven minutes remaining, I carried out my goal: to finish, ideally with all my toenails intact. Mission accomplished. No one can ever take that away from me. Yet science and my body agree: that race was terrible for me. I couldn't run again for a year. Running hurt my feet, my hips, and probably my heart for a time, and my perfectly attached toenails ached for weeks.

Running the marathon without preparation may have been foolish, yet I take pride in the story and do not regret it for a moment. The memory always makes me smile. In my grandfather's 80s, he attributed some of his physical ailments to his high school days pitching and playing football. I asked him, "If you knew then that you were going to suffer this pain now, would you choose not to play?" No way. He loved those days and those memories. There are lots of things that are not good for our bodies. If they bring us joy, we shouldn't rule them out. We have to find the balance and maintenance required so that we can stay as pain-free as possible to continue doing what makes us happy. I'm running again. It's fun and feels normal, if not good. My pace is slower, my distance is shorter, but there is pleasure in the jog.

My inability to feel probably helped me run that race. *Learning to feel* is what helped me recover. Try not to get discouraged when you start something new and don't know what you are feeling. Your body is still sensing something even when you don't notice. Becoming aware hasn't always been pleasant. When I first learned to feel my hamstrings, it was more like a cramp than a rushing feeling of joy, but getting my hamstrings to fire properly has reduced the pain in my knees caused by the running. Ultimately, the emphasis on feeling that I learned from Pilates keeps me running. I notice mild pain sooner, and I can do exercises to help solve the problem so that it doesn't take me out of commission. We don't always have to give up the activities we love that take a toll on our bodies, but we may need to give our bodies more TLC if we want them to continue pushing for us.

In my 20s, I ran six miles a day. When I would go for a hike, by the end of the day, my knees hurt so much that the weight of my pants on my kneecaps made me cringe. Today, over a decade later, I should have more wear and tear on my knees, but they hurt less in general and especially after hiking. Typically, now I run three miles a day, four times a week, and vary my other workouts with Pilates, swimming, yoga, interval training, walking, and kickboxing. I also use trekking poles when I hike a mountain. I listened and learned more about what my body needed to keep me doing activities I didn't want to give up. I get to enjoy all the activities now with less pain. All day there are many movements and senses that our body picks up on that we dismiss. The body is constantly receiving signals and often falling into patterns. To alter patterns for better performance, to reduce pain, or to create superior health, we need to hone in on the signals and feedback our body provides and enact tiny tweaks.

Moving with purpose enhances the movement. You learn about your body, what feels good and what hurts, where your deep strength is, and where you have weaknesses. Learning to feel, with practice and patience, can provide a sense of control. You have to gain awareness of those things before you can make a change. The first step is to notice. Currently, you might be noticing pain. But what else do you feel?

Appreciating Sensation

Ian Waterman, a British man, contracted a rare disease in the '70s that destroyed many, if not all, of the sensory nerves below his neck. He was told he would never walk again; he wasn't paralyzed but couldn't feel or sense himself in space. Using his vision to look at his body and the world around him, he retrained himself to walk. No one understands how. The other people with this disease never made the progress he did. He was disciplined, watched himself, and considered each movement: flex foot, lift leg, pull leg forward, stabilize core, swing arm forward for balance, control descent of leg, engage pelvic stabilizers to balance during transition from one foot to the other. Basic movement that you and I take for granted requires the same effort for him that running a marathon would for us, especially if we had to solve complicated math problems while running. Relearning to walk took time, practice, and patience. He has no way to adjust muscularly for the change in his environment. He said, "If the world were a cricket field, I'd be in heaven, and if the world were a pebbly beach, I'd commit suicide."

Have you ever considered what it would be like to lose your sense of touch and not be able to feel? I find it inconceivable. Imagine if you walked to your car today and stepped on a pebble. Your body would perceive the pebble and adjust without you having to worry about it. It won't make the slightest dent in your day. You would never remember or think about that pebble again. But if you lost sensation in the way Waterman did, that pebble would knock you down. Or if the power went out, you would immediately fall down without any way to see your movement. When you go to sleep tonight and the lights are out, try to imagine what it would be like to be unable to feel yourself in space. It's an ability we take for granted.

At the end of all my Pilates classes, we check our balance. Some people have to step off their one-eighth of an inch rubber mat onto the floor because they feel too wobbly on the mat. The difference is so subtle, but it matters. If you have fairly good balance, you probably would not notice the difference, because our body propriocepts (I just made up a verb) a ton of information without us perceiving the change in sensation. That's what proprioception is. There is a benefit for the body of doing movement on different surfaces like a yoga mat, a carpeted floor, a hardwood floor, the grass, or the sand at the beach. Even if you don't notice a difference or don't feel your muscles being challenged in different ways, your body experiences and recognizes the difference.

Lawrence Williams, a psychologist who studies human behavior and what conscious control we have over our actions, found that people reviewing an individual described on paper (like a resumé) had different opinions about the applicant based on what they were holding.[38] Participants holding a hot beverage regarded the person described differently than someone holding an ice-cold beverage. If they were holding a warmer beverage, they tended to describe the person as more trustworthy. Holding a cold ice pack made people more likely to select a gift for themselves over someone else. Without being aware of it, our opinion of a person, a movie, or almost anything else is altered by sensations stimulating our body in that moment: temperature, the weight of an object, the firmness of a chair. The slightest change in our physical world can affect how we think, but most of the time we ignore our sensations. Generally, we seem to have minimal control over how our exteroception, proprioception, and interoception dictate our thoughts. Still, we think we are reasonably rational actors.

The feelings that we get from inside our body contribute to our disposition, our stress level, and our mood. Interoception may influence self-control. A study led by Beate Herbert at the University of Tuebingen in Germany looked at 49 women. Those with more cardiac awareness (the ability to acknowledge accurate heartbeats without taking a pulse) also had more gastric awareness.[39] They noticed when they were full faster and consumed less water than women who had poor cardiac awareness. While we don't need to feel every heartbeat all day long, having a better connection with our inner sense of self could benefit our decisions and our ability for restraint. Today, stop and reflect on one simple thing you take for granted normally. Maybe it's the

---

38 Lawrence E. Williams and John A. Bargh, "Experiencing Physical Warmth Promotes Interpersonal Warmth," *Science* 322, no. 5901 (Oct 2008): 606–7, http://doi.org/10.1126/science.1162548.
39 Beate M. Herbert and Olga Pollatos, "The Body in the Mind: On the Relationship Between Interoception and Embodiment," *Topics in Cognitive Science* 4, no. 4 (Oct 2012): 692–704, https://doi.org/10.1111/j.1756-8765.2012.01189.x.

sunrise or your ability to pour yourself a cup of coffee without thinking about it. Become aware of what you feel physically while pouring that cup or watching that sun rise. Be amazed. Your ability to feel is awe-inspiring. And, someday, it might be the very thing that saves your life. Chances are it already has.

Restorative Sleep

Sleep is imperative for healing, tissue repair, and recovery. Good sleep reduces stress and weight gain, both of which can exacerbate pain. A good night's sleep helps our immune system fight disease, which matters even more if pain is related to autoimmune disease. As we age, we produce less and less human growth hormone (HGH), which the body makes when asleep to help build and repair muscles. Lack of sleep creates a potentially vicious cycle of exhaustion and limited healing.

In addition, multiple hormones affect how we sleep, recover, and feel pain. Lisa Christian, a clinical health psychologist at Ohio State University has linked higher cortisol levels (the stress hormone) with slower wound healing.[40] Though chronic pain and wounds are different, both require time to heal and repair. Our cortisol levels are meant to drop in the evening when we sleep. If we do not get the hours or quality sleep that we require or have high cortisol levels in the evening hours, it could impede healing. Inflammation, common with pain and disease, is also known to inhibit quality sleep.[41] Certain cytokines (proteins in the body) help regulate sleep and inflammation.[42] In the case of chronic pain, these cytokines may reduce the pain threshold and

---

40 Lisa M. Christian et al., "Stress and Wound Healing," *Neuroimmunomodulation* 13, no. 5–6 (2006): 337–46, http://doi.org/10.1159/000104862.
41 Mark R. Zielinski, "Sleep and Inflammation—Intimate Partners in Health and Functioning," Thrive Global, May 16, 2017, https://medium.com/thrive-global/the-fascinating-link-between-inflammation-and-sleep-9d57c2eca013.
42 Tuck Sleep, "Cytokines, Sleep Regulation and Immune Response," updated February 5, 2018, https://www.tuck.com/cytokines/.

be part of an increased pain cycle in the body, similar to how some people taking opioids experience increased pain.[43]

All this information is very daunting, and long nights can feel very lonely, but you're not alone. According to the Centers for Disease Control and Prevention (CDC), about a quarter of people living in the United States self-report having a sleep disorder (that's about 80 million people). The National Institute of Neurological Disorders and Strokes estimates 40 million Americans have a chronic sleep disorder and 20 million have an occasional sleep disorder resulting in $16 billion in medical costs each year. Those figures are not a peaceful way to lull you to sleep, but when sleep deprivation has you panicked, know that you and 80 million other people are awake.

My mom and grandma are constantly apologizing to me for my inability to sleep. They think they genetically cursed me. My OBGYN once referred to my inability to sleep as "the curse of the woman." Instead of blaming Grandma, blame Thomas Edison for any trouble you have sleeping. The invention of the light bulb has thrown off our natural sleep cycle. The hormone melatonin influences our sleep and is linked to dark and light. It rises with nightfall to help us fall asleep and lowers during the day when the sun is shining. But in our world of artificial light we stay up later and find ourselves groggy in the morning because melatonin is still present. Camping can create a more regulated melatonin level that matches sunrise and sunset. One study found that campers tended to go to bed earlier and get up earlier, and even though they were rising early, they felt less groggy.[44] Their sleep habits synchronized with natural light, and

---

43 Goeij, Moniek et al, "Systematic Inflammation Decreases Pain Threshold in Humans in Vivo," PLOS ONE 8 no. 12 (2013), https://doi.org/10.1371/journal.pone.0084159.
44 Joel N. Shurkin,"Trouble Sleeping? Go Camping," *Scientific American*, August 2, 2013.

their melatonin levels were lower in the mornings compared to mornings when they were not camping.

Historically, our ancestors woke up in the middle of the night between their "first" and "second" sleep. They didn't keep to the eight-hour sleep cycle we've adopted but rather slept with the dark, sleeping longer hours in the winter. It was typical to sleep for about four hours and then to be active for an hour or two before falling back to sleep for another four or so hours. In their middle-of-the-night break, they didn't lie awake hemming and hawing. They read, wrote, prayed, visited neighbors, had sex (a 16th century doctor's manual suggested that after first sleep was the best time to conceive). In the 1990s, a physiatrist led an experiment where he created a 14-hour night situation; over the course of a month, participants developed our ancestors' sleeping patterns: sleeping for four hours, waking up for one to two hours, and falling back to sleep for four hours.[45]

We put pressure on ourselves to conform to a sleep cycle which may not be natural for us. On top of that, we no longer exist in an environment that cues our hormones to operate optimally. But alarms and electricity aren't going away. Those eight hours at night may be the only time we have to sleep. The good news is aerobic exercise does help us sleep. Find any tip that provides you better sleep: dark room, no electronics, cool temperatures, a pleasurable nighttime routine, warm feet, melatonin (talk to your doctor first), counting sheep or breaths. You can even try positive self-talk, telling yourself, "I am the best sleeper in the whole world." Try anything, no matter how silly (though be cautious of anything that costs money). It doesn't matter how peculiar your tactics are. If they work for you, they work.

---

45 Stephanie Hegarty, "The Myth of the Eight-Hour Sleep," *BBC News*, February 22, 2012.

CHAPTER 6: LAYING THE GROUNDWORK

The body is an integrative whole. Our daily activities, food choices, exercises, and moods influence our body constantly. Exercise is an important tool in feeling and being healthy. We need it, especially in our sedentary world. That being said, it is unrealistic to assume that one hour of exercise every day will unravel eight hours in a chair. Even if our day isn't spent in a chair, however we spend most of our time will start to be reflected in the body. The changes we need to make to reduce pain need to happen throughout the entire day in addition to the exercises we make time for.

Considering your body in space throughout the day can help you feel better. Check in at different moments. If your back hurts when you are doing something, is there a simple change you can make to relieve the pain? If your neck hurts, can you make a subtle adjustment? Perhaps it's the chair or the bucket seat in your car causing your discomfort. Maybe if you get up and do two gentle stretches or walk around the office for as little as five minutes, the pain diminishes. This section of the book is intended to encourage you to consider your body throughout the day, not just when you are consciously moving.

Posture

For the sake of our strained bodies, we must discuss where good posture should begin. It's sadly not as simple as sticking our chest out and pulling our shoulders down like many of us were taught. Posture is defined as "a position of a person's body when standing or sitting" or "a particular way of dealing with or considering something, an approach or an attitude." When talking about the body, we tend to discuss definition number one, the actual physical position of our body. While that's important and does relate to our physical well-being, the second definition is directly linked to the first. Think of mopey Eeyore from Winnie the Pooh. He is depressed, and you can see it in his whole being: his body sags, his head slumps, his movement is slow. He is miserable, and we know before he even opens his mouth that we are about to witness a whine and a mope. Our posture is the first impression we give to the world and often dictates how people view us.

Remember when you were kid and you'd have a fight with your parents about the clothes you were wearing and what people would think? Dress as a goth or a hippie and people will prejudge. Dress in a short skirt and people might prejudge. We debate if any judgement is right or wrong, fair or appropriate, but it happens, and we know it does. If clothes make the man, posture makes the person.

Our posture is like our attire. It changes our attitude and the perceived attitude of those who encounter us throughout the day. For example, the Wonder Woman posture has been shown to increase confidence and enhance performance, particularly before walking into a stressful situation.[46] Next time you have a big event, go into a bathroom stall (where no one can see you) and make yourself larger than life, pushing your hands up to the ceiling and puffing your chest out, or standing tall and firm with your hands on your hips for two minutes. Try it and see for yourself how you feel afterward.

On a biological level, posture influences our stress and hormone levels, which have important implications for pain. Since stress can increase pain sensations, reducing or mitigating stress levels can be an important aspect of pain prevention and management. A team of researchers at the University of Pittsburg led by Peter Stick, PhD, discovered that posture and core strength are intricately linked with stress levels and adrenal function based on the massive neural network that connect both to the brain. This was a shock to the researchers, as they suspected there might be one or two connections between the cerebral cortex and the adrenal medulla (which regulates stress hormones in the body). While they are not sure how many connections there actually are, in addition to showing a significant association that may prove the mind-body connection, Stick's team uncovered that neural pathways connecting the brain to the adrenals are intertwined with the axial motor cortex (the part of the brain that controls the muscles in your core or trunk).[47] The portion of the brain that plans and initiates movement also links to your adrenal medulla, indicating that movement of the core and posture are intricately connected with the release of stress hormones. Yoga and Pilates may be good for reducing stress and pain, not only because of

46 David Biello, "Inside the Debate About Power Posing: A Q&A with Amy Cuddy," Ideas.Ted.com, February 22, 2017, https://ideas.ted.com/inside-the-debate-about-power-posing-a-q-a-with-amy-cuddy/.
47 University of Pittsburgh Medical Center, "Pitt Research Provides New Insights into How the Mind Influences the Body," August 15, 2016, https://www.upmc.com/media/NewsReleases/2016/Pages/strick-stress-research.aspx.

their meditative properties, but because they move the muscles of the core, ideally in a way that improves postural muscles. The findings from this research were so compelling that Stick, the lead scientist on these studies, started attending Pilates classes. (A neuroscientist who does Pilates is my idea of an incredible leading man. A TV show must be in production already.)

Generations have all been told not to slump or slouch. As a society, we have made posture important. But what should our posture look like for optimal health? What are indicators of good posture? Your posture changes from day-to-day and week-to-week. We all have postural tendencies, which can change quickly or over time. Sometimes when people begin Pilates with me, they ask if Pilates will make them taller. Pilates won't make the bones of your legs longer, but it does teach you how to hold yourself with good posture and alignment. That change may provide a higher reading on a doctor's chart. Gravity had been winning the long game, pushing down on your body. Pilates taught you how to take advantage of the height you always had.

My friend Chris and his family went to a lakeside cabin in upstate New York every year when he was growing up. Recently, he went to the cabin with his brothers, and they compared themselves to the marks on the wall where his mother had recorded their heights over time. He took his photograph beside his height markers. At nearly age 70, he was two inches shorter than the last time his height was recorded at age 16. Nothing in the body is constant, including posture and alignment. Your posture may be different when you wake up, after a long car ride, or after a fitness class. It is certainly different decade from decade.

When we picture perfect posture, Leonardo Di Vinci's *Vitruvian Man* comes to mind. It's the depiction of perfect proportions.

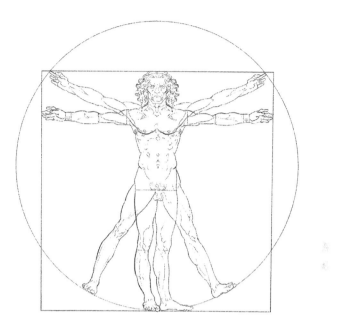

I have yet to meet a person who is perfectly symmetrical. We are all a little longer, more crooked, or slightly twisted on one side compared to the other. Our liver is on one side, and our heart isn't centered. We should not force everyone into a perfectly square box or circle where they fit just so. Perfection is not our goal when thinking about posture. Comfort is the goal. Poor posture leads to pain. If you can find a position that relieves you of strain, that is your good postural position for now. It may change in the future. We can use plumb lines and boxes and angles as tools to help us find a good posture, but none of us are exactly the same. There is no steadfast rule.

Maintaining an upright posture is surprisingly hard work. Gravity is a relentless opponent. What we need to consider is whether all our bones, joints, and spaces line up with each other. Consider the major landmarks of the body. Generally, our ankles, hips, ribs and head should all line up one over the other. The pelvis should not jut forward while the ribs sway back. We refer to those big, boney parts as masses. In between them should be natural curves or spaces (your neck, low back, behind the knees). If any of the masses are sticking out in front or back, they put strain on the spaces. Good posture will create space where there needs to be space. For example, when our posture is aligned, all the muscles around the shoulder can move freely without impingement. There would be relative balance between the front and back or the sides of the body. Tension and pressure would be somewhat equal from side to side and front to back. We would not have more weight on one leg or kick our hip out to the side. Start to think of the positions you put your body in all day long whether standing, sitting, or in motion.

Can you find a neutral place in your body where you feel comfortable, where basic movement like standing or walking becomes effortless? All joints and curves in the spine have a neutral, and everyone's neutral can be different. Finding yours may take some experimenting. Thinking about where your parts are in space and where they are related to one another can be a daily exercise that helps alleviate pain.

Common Postural Faux Pas

One of the most common faulty postures, known as a swayback, occurs when the pelvis swings forward, and to counterbalance that so as not to fall forward, the ribs swing back. To counterbalance the ribs, the head juts out. If you are ever washing dishes or your hands and notice your pelvis is pushing into the sink or counter top, you probably have your hips too far forward. Try stacking your ribs and hips one on top of the other, masses over masses. Our head usually sticks out forward of the rest of our body. This is to counteract that forward slump in the mid-back and shoulder of the swayback posture. We need to think of pulling it back, but this can feel uncomfortable. To correct this, we must first work on that slump or it will be really hard to find a comfortable place for the neck to exist.

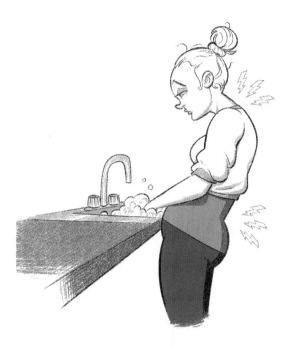

Many of us also tend to slouch forward, caving in at the ribs and rounding the shoulders forward. Then we are told to have better posture and so stick our chest out by shoving our ribs forward and squeezing our shoulder blades together. This correction does not create a sense of neutral anywhere in our spine or shoulders. Adjusting for the slouch in our upper backs is perhaps the hardest to adjust accurately. Instead of sticking your chest out and tugging your shoulders down, think of getting long from your tailbone to the crown of your head. Imagine creating space between each vertebra in your back. Get longer anywhere you can. Imagine your sternum (breastbone) getting longer. Instead of moving your breastbone forward, think of pulling the bottom of the breastbone down and the top up. It will not feel like a big move. The bone can't actually get longer, but you can create more space around it. Once you feel like your breastbone is as long as it can get from end to end, think of your collarbones getting longer out to the sides.

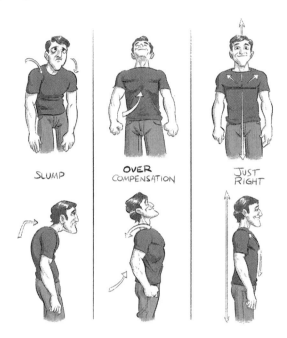

Picture a dot in the center of your breastbone with arrows radiating out in all directions. You get long from top to bottom, but also sideways out of both shoulders. It's not easy, but it will improve your posture and balance your muscles better than the easier move of jutting the ribs out.

Change is not all or nothing. Just because you read this today does not mean that for the rest of your life you have to keep your head in perfect alignment. It is always a balancing act, and trying to change too much too fast could cause other problems. We look to altering alignment to help reduce pain, but we don't want to get so overwhelmed by perfect stature that we lose natural, free-flowing movement. The emphasis should be on how the movement feels and what makes us feel better. We want control and to be able to stabilize on command and move fluidly on command. We are seeking comfort, ease, and balance in our structure as with everything else in the body.

While the suggestions above consider misalignment from front to back, we can have poor posture from side to side. Do you regularly catch yourself standing with one hip kicked out to the side? Is it always the same hip? Try shifting your weight into your other hip for a while. Try keeping equal weight on both feet with neither hip kicked out. Practice whenever you get stuck in line somewhere. Play with the balance of your weight between your feet. Do you find parts of your body working harder than others? Do you feel tension anywhere? Is your butt or are your quads engaged or squeezing? Can you relax any muscles without falling over? Make this a game, and suddenly standing in line is no longer wasted time. In fact, if you ever get stuck waiting anywhere and your body is with you, you never need to feel like time is wasted again.

Play. The body is a big experiment, and it's different every day. But if you want to get out of chronic pain, you need to check in with how it is feeling and what it is doing often. Notice a habit, and alter that habit to feel better. For a visual sense of what is going on with your posture, ask a friend to take four photos of you. Kick off your shoes. Wear whatever you want, but a tank top and shorts will make it easier to see your own joints. Don't try to stand with good posture. Be honest and stand in your natural, typical slouch. Then have your friend take a picture of you from the front, back, and both sides. Your body can change day-to-day and hour-to-hour, so this is not perfect, but it is a helpful guide. Here are illustrations made from my actual pictures.

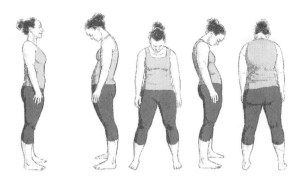

Even if you are not an expert on the human body, you can probably notice that something is wrong with my neck when you see these illustrations.

It seems to have given up. I know this is a problem area for me, so I try to notice when I can hold my neck differently. For instance, I tend to look at my feet while walking, so I make an effort to look straight ahead and keep my chin parallel to the ground. Or instead of looking down at my phone, sometimes I raise it to eye level, encouraging my neck to hold my noggin up. It takes conscious thought and physical effort for me to hold my head up, but when I think of it, I do it. Compare how different my posture looks when I make an effort versus when I resort to bad habits.

Breathe Better

"Smile, breathe, and go slowly."

—Thich Nhat Hanh

Breathing. We do it without even thinking about it 12 to 20 times per minute. We do it to relax or to give ourselves energy, filling our lungs with about 11,000 liters of air every day. It seems so simple, yet many of us are not breathing to our fullest potential and that means we aren't fueling our bodies to our fullest potential. The good news is that we have the ability to alter our breath pattern instantly.

Take a second now to breathe as normally as you can. I know once you start focusing on your breath, it's never really normal, but try. Take a couple of breaths and notice where you breathe naturally. Are you a belly breather? A rib breather? Do your shoulders move up and down? Can you not tell the difference? Do you feel like you naturally take a deep breath or a shallow breath? Do you breathe through your nose or your mouth? Then time yourself for a minute. How many breaths do you take in one minute? Note what stands out to you while you are breathing.

The body breathes spontaneously, even if we increase activity. We don't think about breathing more frequently or heavily. The body adjusts based on its need for oxygen. But one thing is a guarantee: breathing always involves movement, and that movement involves lots of muscles. One of the functions of your pelvic floor muscles is to aid in respiration. If you pee a little when you cough, sneeze, or do a jumping jack, you are completely normal, but it does mean muscles aren't firing properly or they lack the necessary tone to fire. You can restore muscle tone. A healthy pelvic floor keeps us from wetting ourselves when we have a hearty belly laugh, because the strength and endurance of your pelvic floor matters when you breathe.

When you breathe generally, and definitely when you take a deep breath, you should be working muscles in your neck, all the muscles around your ribs, back muscles, shoulder muscles, abdominal muscles, and the muscles at the base of your pelvis. If it's connected to your ribs, it's moving. When you experience pain, consider a few deep breaths. As long as you are not suffering from a rib injury, even if every other movement hurts, breathing is still an option. Inhaling oxygenates the muscles. Breathing fuels our body for movement and is one of the micro-movements we can use to reduce pain.

Though our body breathes intuitively, we can adjust our breathing to alter our voice, sing, meditate, adjust our mood, change our tension level, activate organs, sync breath with movement, or increase a stretch. Breathing is versatile. Our mind and muscles have a lot of control over our breath when we want them to. While breathing can cause movement in any part of the trunk, the air only goes in the lungs. Still, everything else has to move around to provide room for the expansion of the lungs. Our shoulders may rise, our ribs should expand. The abdominal muscles extend. The pelvic floor, or Kegel muscles, descend on a deep inhale. At rest, like reading or watching TV, you exchange about a half liter of air per breath. When you increase the quantity needed, whether intentionally or in the case where you get winded going for a run, people on average can fit anywhere from two and a half to three liters of air in their lungs.

Tom Sietas set the record for longest static apnea (the fancy term for holding your breath) at 22 minutes and 22 seconds.

The diaphragm is a dome-shaped muscle (actually two muscles, one on each side) at the base of our ribcage that separates our lungs from the organs, intestines, and stomach beneath. This muscle contracts concentrically (shortening) when we inhale, pulling downward and providing space for our lungs to expand. A lazy, lax diaphragm can result in acid reflux, a problem plaguing 20 percent of the population. If your chronic pain is indigestion, you might want to consider some breathing exercises.

Hopefully, you are not sick of hearing about the transversus abdominis (TA). In fact, I hope those two letters are music to your ears, inspiring the same feelings as seeing an old friend who, no matter how much time passes, ensures you that you have a true, trusted, dependable companion. The TA and the diaphragm may be best friends. While it has generally been determined that the TA is vital to spinal stability, there is less research linking the diaphragm and the spine even though the two are attached. However, that is slowly changing. A review investigating how breathing exercises reduce back pain found that depending on the technique, certain breathing exercises could be as effective if not more effective than physical therapy for treating chronic, non-specific low back pain.[48] Another study that compared the associations between body mass index, physical activity, incontinence, and respiratory disorders in young, mid-age, and older-aged women with back pain, found that incontinence and allergies had the strongest correlation with back pain among all age groups. Respiratory disorders (asthma, allergies, and sinusitis) correlated with back pain in mid-age and older women. The results indicate that pelvic floor stability, breathing, and a functional diaphragm may be more related to back pain than obesity.[49] In other words, your core muscles—the TA, pelvic floor, and multifidi (the small muscles between the vertebrae in the spine)—working with the diaphragm may be a major factor in unwinding low back pain. The good news is that breathing is free. The challenging news is that some people find deep breathing exercises very difficult. But there is hope and potential in these findings.

---

48 Barton E. Anderson and K. C. H. Bliven, "The Use of Breathing Exercises in Treatment of Chronic, Nonspecific Low Back Pain," Journal of Sport Rehabilitation 26 no. 5 (2017): 452–58, https://doi.org/10.1123/jsr.2015-0199.

49 M. D. Smith et al, "Disorders of Breathing and Continence Have a Stronger Association with Back Pain than Obesity and Physical Activity," Australian Journal of Physiotherapy 52, no. 1 (2006): 11–16, https://doi.org/10.1016/S0004-9514(06)70057-5.

The zone of apposition (ZOA) is the space where the dome-shaped diaphragm can move. The proper tone of your TA and other abdominal muscles, like the obliques, determine the size of the ZOA and the tension in the diaphragm. Optimal space in the ZOA may help you breathe better and reduce back pain, allowing the diaphragm to act as a spine stabilizer. The TA and diaphragm constantly work in harmony, like yin and yang. When you inhale, the diaphragm shortens while the TA lengthens. They do the opposite on exhalation. Every breath involves these two muscles dancing as partners. When working properly, this is effortless, but dysfunction of one can limit the other and cause problems throughout the body. Stop and breathe for a second and picture a partnership between your abdominals and diaphragm, like a flowing wave on each breath. Envision the body working together with a goal of healing.

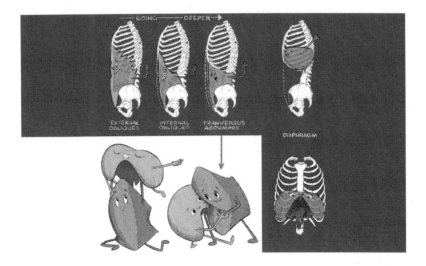

Different types of movement benefit from different breathing styles. There are many ways to take a breath: belly breathing, yoga breathing, Pilates breathing, Lamaze. Each style utilizes a different depth, rhythm, orifice, and direction to propel the air. One is not better than the other. It's like all movement: variety is key. You can take deep relaxing breaths that slowly engage most of the muscles of the trunk or short staccato breaths that really work the muscles of the neck. You can breathe through your nose or your mouth, one nostril or both. Breathing through the nose enables your nose hairs to filter the air and keep the throat from drying out.

The ribcage and muscles involved with inhalation become more limber and flexible with practice, so you can increase your capacity to take in air. By strengthening muscles of expiration, you enhance your ability to rid yourself of "old" air. Breathing is a release—a letting go—so if something doesn't feel good, never force yourself or feel stressed about it. Notice it. If you are used to a shallow breath, learning to take a deep breath can be frustrating. Getting frustrated makes the task more daunting. Try again another day. You can always try something that hasn't worked in the past and find success in the future. I like to tell my clients, "It doesn't have to be perfect until next week. Same rule applies next week." We are seeking progress, not perfection.

Breathing Exercises

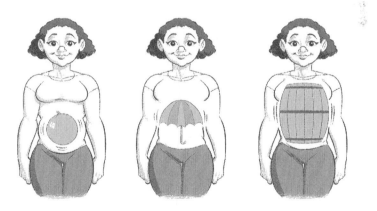

Many of us take for granted how important and how helpful breathing can be to unwind pain, heal, and help us calm down.

Often breathing is an area where people get really frustrated. When doing these exercises, try to judge yourself less and explore what you feel.

Belly Breath. As you breathe, let your stomach extend like a balloon inflating on each inhale. Then exhale drawing the navel toward the spine, pushing all the air up and out. Try to notice the abdominals and the pelvic floor expanding to let air in and engaging to help push air out.

Pilates Lateral Breath. Breathe into the sides and back of the ribs, trying to keep the lower abdominals gently engaged (grain of salt here). Imagine your ribs opening up like an umbrella or an accordion on the inhale. On the exhale, visualize your ribs close down toward your spine. This is a challenging place to send the breath and not normal for most of us. Consider trying it lying down, knees bent, feet on the floor. Having the floor beneath you may help you feel the breath going into the back of your ribs.

3-D Breath. Try to expand your trunk in every direction: front to back, side to side, top to bottom like a barrel. How much of your trunk can you actually feel expand?

Staccato Breath. Take five quick, short breaths in through your nose followed by five quick short breaths out your mouth. Repeat five to ten times. If you feel light-headed, stop. You should feel the muscles of your neck get more involved. If you can't sense that, place your fingertips gently on your neck to physically feel the activity.

Counting Breath. Assume a comfortable position (seated or lying on the floor knees bent). Take a normal breath for you. Then inhale for a count of four. Exhale for four. Inhale for five. Exhale for five. Keep repeating, adding a second to each breath, and learn how many seconds you can inhale and exhale for. I've met people who can get all the way to 30 seconds. Tip: on the inhale, since you will be taking in more air each time, focus on breathing in slowly.

Start with these exercises because they are simple, but feel free to get creative and make up your own breathing pattern. What calms you down? What feels good when you are sore somewhere? What helps you sleep? Maybe you always prefer to link breathing with movement. Pick a simple move like a head nod or pointing and flexing your feet to sync with your breath. If it feels good, it's not wrong.

Mindfulness

Mindfulness and mindset matter. It's better to move while distracted than not to move at all. But if you intend to build strength faster while reducing injury, it's time to pay attention. If you want to change a neuromuscular deficiency, you need the nerves and muscles to work together to form a memorable modification. That may take some thinking. This can be especially hard in our super-tech, super-speed, multitask-driven world. Our current world requires that we check in with our bodies even more. I say this as someone who is terrible and uncommitted to meditation or mindfulness. It's not easy. I fight meditation, don't enjoy it, think I'm bad at it, and pretty much never want to do it. Still, it is extremely valuable. Research proves it is. But, if like me, you are turned off by meditation, there are many other ways to be mindful.

Years ago, I read *The Art of Happiness: A Handbook for Living* by the Dalai Lama and Howard C. Cutler, MD, and, to be honest, I found it frustrating. In my memory (though it has been years since I read it), a single mom working multiple jobs to support her family asked how she was supposed to find time for meditation. The Dalai Lama's response was basically that she had to. There was no excuse. (Totally paraphrased here, but that was the gist as I understood it.) I was so annoyed for the woman and decided the Dalai Lama was out of touch. Not long after, I read the book *The Miracle of Mindfulness: An Introduction to the Practice of Meditation* by Thich Nhat Hanh, a Vietnamese Buddhist monk. When asked basically the same question, he responded that we all should attempt to be more present and start to recognize the importance of the mundane tasks we sometimes resent. If you are washing dishes, instead of thinking about everything else you have to do, focus on washing the dishes, recognizing how important and essential clean dishes are for you and your family. If you can't wash a teacup, you can't have tea. And if you can't be aware of yourself while washing the pot, what are the chances you will be in the moment when you are drinking the tea?

Hanh writes, "I clean this teapot with the kind of attention I would have were I giving the baby Buddha or Jesus a bath." Whatever task lies before you, that specific moment is as valuable as any moment you may have, so try to give it your undivided attention. I would add to his theory of mindfulness that you would benefit by noting the physical sensations of what you are doing. How does the water feel? How do the soap suds sensate? Is the teapot smooth, gritty, oily, greasy? On the one hand, noticing these sensations is important so that you can be present, but if you are in pain, beginning to notice all the sensations your body feels is the start of helping your nervous system unwind. Paying attention to sensations can also tune you in to noticing pain incrementally so that you can catch it early.

Being Aware Can Lead to Beneficial Change

We typically don't put emphasis on what we physically feel throughout the day. We notice when pain gets in the way, like when our neck or back aches. But if we practiced mindfulness regularly, we might notice a problem early on and be able to stop it from becoming excruciating. We also might notice that there is a good deal of time that we actually feel good, a sensation often taken for granted. It's peculiar that we take our sense of touch for granted because physical perception is probably our most important sensation. Without it, we would truly feel lost in our own world.

We can find time for mindfulness in our daily tasks, but we can also be mindful in movement. Start very simply. If you take a fitness class, begin by being aware. Does a particular motion hurt anywhere in your body? Does your hip pop and click when you move it on certain exercises? Why? Is there anything you can change that takes the discomfort away? Ask yourself whether you feel the exercise where the movement is intended. In other words, do you feel squats in your quads and glutes? If you are doing an abdominal exercise, do you feel your abs working or is your neck straining? Can you adjust something about the way you are doing the movement so that the neck stops hurting? Finding the right spot or angle may take practice and time. Learn to be okay with that. Change does not happen in an instant. In addition to asking an instructor for guidance, ask yourself. You know your body better than anyone. If you experiment and listen to the feedback your body gives you, you can sometimes find the best place all by yourself. You know what to do even if you don't realize it yet.

Making a change in your body is like any other skill: you have to practice and pay attention. You would never have aced a test in school if you didn't start by listening to the lecture. Everything you do, including moving, without mindfulness is diminished. When you aren't present, you devalue the moment. I don't say that as a judgement or an expectation that you will always be mindful. Today, I walked into the pharmacy frustrated, tense, distracted, and aggravated for no good reason. I waited in line in a huff, requested my medicine, and was informed my medication would be ready next week. "Please double check," I asked. "I pick it up the same time every month."

As it turns out, I'd shown up a week early. Frazzled and feeling foolish, when they asked for my birthday, I stumbled. I had forgotten the simplest question. My delay lasted about three seconds, leaving my pharmacist to ask if it was a tough question. "It shouldn't be," I responded. Then I paid for something else, turned around, and walked into a free-standing sign notifying others to stay back for privacy. "Oh, excuse me," I announced in a booming voice before recognizing the sign wasn't another human being. The pharmacist, the next person in line, and I all laughed. The laughter brought me back to the present. More often than not, laughter always works. Who doesn't want to be in the moment for a chuckle or a shared smile?

If the end result of distraction was laughter, then that's a good ending. We need to expect that there are moments during the day we will fade into the recesses of our mind. Still, we need to encourage time to be mindful, notice the mundane, and check in with our own body.

Mindful Multitaskers

We are competent multitaskers. Our body can function without being present. Think of how many times you've driven somewhere only to realize you spent the whole trip on autopilot. Still, now and then it's beneficial to check in with your body. Maybe if you focus on how you walk or how you breathe, you will discover something. Do you walk with a really heavy foot and pound down the hallway? Do you have a click in your hips now and again on certain steps? Is there something you can change about your everyday movement that will make you feel better, move with more ease, or engage more muscles?

Adjusting bad habits requires mindfulness. And if you suffer from chronic pain, you probably have developed a bad habit over time, a habit that resulted in the pain or developed out of how you altered the body in response to the pain. If you are working on corrective exercises or going to physical or occupational therapy, mindfulness and paying attention become vital for success. Regularly practicing mindfulness-based stress reductions lessens back pain in women.[50] Making a change in your body is like any other skill: it requires repetition, focus, and time.

We can be mindful about the way we sit, stand, walk, and breathe. That mindfulness can create positive changes in our body. Forming a new habit is hard, so find reminders to think about it. Every time you see a stop sign, red light, doorknob, remote control, or microwave, practice the new habit you are trying to imprint on your brain. Give yourself visual cues throughout the day that remind you to think of how you are holding yourself in space. You can change your body, so check in with yourself regularly to make change. One place to start is taking note of when you become distracted and learning to redirect your attention. As adults, we no longer have to take comprehension quizzes to ensure we are paying attention and prove competency of material. Be aware if you are distracted when reading, talking, or working on any project. What is distracting you, and how can you bring yourself back?

If you are in a position to schedule regular meditation in your life, that is wonderful. If it's not up your alley, you may benefit from experimenting with calming the mind once in a while. Vegetables are good for us even if we don't always like them.

---

50 Sudha Banth and Maryam Didehdar Ardebil, "Effectiveness of Mindfulness Meditation on Pain and Quality of Life of Patients with Chronic Low Back Pain," *International Journal of Yoga* 8, no. 2 (Jul–Dec 2015): 128–33, https://www.ncbi. nlm.nih.gov/pmc/articles/PMC4479890/.

Scientific evidence bolsters the benefits of meditation, and there are many varieties you can try. When I was in college, I used to run six miles a day, usually by myself, and I thought of it as meditation. Some days, I'd get great ideas for papers or problems I was trying to sort out. I still stand by that as a form of meditation even though it is not traditional.

However, if you know you won't commit to 30, 20, even 5 minutes a day of dedicated meditation, would stopping at random times throughout the day work for you? Might you do something kind for your body or mind every day? That might mean going for a walk or taking a bath. Thinking of holding better posture or walking with a softer step might be the thing for you. Even if you only start with 30 seconds, any starting place is better than none.

Tips for How Mindfulness Can Help You Heal

Put distractions away

We live in a world that is more distracting than ever, filled with TVs, phones, computers, and fully booked schedules. No matter where we turn, we are bombarded with something else we should or could be doing. Is there a weeknight that everyone in your house would agree to unplug? Play a game? Sit and read? Go for a walk? If you feel overwhelmed throughout the week, think of an activity that gave you pleasure before cell phones made us constantly connected. Maybe it was taking a walk or going to the movies. Maybe it was listening to music while sprawled out on your bed. Whatever pops in your head, try to carve out time for that activity once a month, even if it's only for 20 minutes. If it doesn't provide the same joy you remember, find a new pleasure.

Get outside

Take a walk or a run without technology. Breathe in the air. Look at the trees. Studies suggest that when people exercise outdoors, they walk faster but say it feels easier. Environment can be a motivator to move. Outdoor workouts in "green space"—a place with a trail, park, or greenery—boosts mood and self-esteem.[51] Add "blue space" with a view of water and parks to provide even more benefit.

Check in

At some point every day, try to stop for a moment and notice what you feel, emotionally and physically. Does your body feel good or bad? Do you feel good, bad, happy, sad, tense, excited? Our body is constantly giving us signals about how we feel, and if we never stop and listen, something minor can develop into something major.

You may surprise yourself and find that you feel better than you expected. You'll come to appreciate days you feel really good. Once when I was going through a difficult time, I felt like an emotional disaster. My boyfriend, who didn't think I was that bad, recommended that I mark the calendar each day with a happy, sad, or flat face. Drawing the emoticon took seconds at the end of the day. By the end of the month, I looked back and had mostly good days with maybe only three to five sad or flat faces. It changed my perspective because I was feeling like those three somber days were the majority. They weren't. Pain and sadness can be so powerful that they seem to overrun the good days. Stop to notice, and you may discover things aren't as catastrophic as they seem when life is whizzing by in a whir.

---

51 BBC News, "'Green' Exercise Quickly 'Boosts Mental Health,'" Updated May 1, 2010.

Be aware of what you put on and in your body

When you have pain, the food you eat may contribute. Consider keeping a journal to see if anything in particular seems to increase your arthritis or other pain. Then it is up to you whether you cut that from your diet. You can make the choice to eat something even if you know it may increase pain while also making a plan to anticipate and deal with the pain.

Also, consider everything that touches your body: shoes, belts, handbags, beds, office desks, couches, bucket car seats, and dining room chairs. A few years ago, I had an ache in my low back that wouldn't go away. Movement would ease it momentarily, but it persisted. I'd been dealing with the problem for a couple months when I went to visit my best friend, Julie, in Chicago (the same Julie who threw the infamous Peter Pan birthday party). Before my arrival, she mentioned filling our days with intense physical activity. I told her that would be unlikely, since my back was limiting my movement.

Julie's decade-old bed was like sleeping on a cloud, softer than a bed of cotton balls. This is not the kind of bed I'd pick for myself. I like a firm, supportive mattress. Yet, somehow after one night in her bed, I woke up with zero back pain. Somewhat skeptically through the entire workout we did the next morning, I waited for the pain to return. We rode bikes around Chicago all afternoon the next day. Through all our revelries, my back was fine. I flew home, and the next morning getting out of my own bed made me feel like I'd aged 50 years overnight. "It's the bed," I yawned.

Apparently, when it comes to sleeping, I am the living version of the Princess and the Pea or Goldilocks (pick your favorite fictional character who has trouble finding the perfect bed). Our bed was fairly new, so I had never considered that my mattress might be the culprit in my pain. If your bed is the problem, spending one night at a friend's house or a hotel should help you find out. I wouldn't invest in a new bed until you have evidence your bed is the offender.

We take for granted how much our bed, pillow, and shoes, can affect how we feel, but we spend a lot of time sleeping in beds and walking in shoes. Consider everything, from the way your clothes fit to the shape of your desk chair. It all might be altering your body, and those can be very easy (though not always cheap) fixes.

Hug a good friend

Physical connection can literally change your body. Couples who have positive conversations and loving physical interactions (a tender touch or a snuggle) have faster wound healing.[52] According to a University of North Carolina study, hugging for 20 seconds releases oxytocin and lowers blood pressure in women.[53] Oxytocin has been deemed our "cuddle chemical" or the "hug hormone," and is related to comfort and bonding. Chronic musculoskeletal pain is not the same as a wound, but I'd gamble that good relationships help relieve chronic pain in much the same way. Human contact from someone we love helps us heal. Since learning this, Matt will sometimes grab me, especially after a tough day, and announce, "It's time for your dose of oxytocin." Then he hugs me. It works. I'm not sure how he regulates the specific dose, but connection with another living being diminishes pain, both physical and emotional.

---

52 Jean-Philippe Gouin et al., "Marital Behavior, Oxytocin, Vasopressin, and Wound Healing," *Psychoneuroendocrinology* 35, no. 7 (2010): 1082–90, https://doi.org/10.1016/j.psyneuen.2010.01.009.
53 Jan McColm, "A Hug a Day," *Endeavors*, UNC-Chapel Hill, January 1, 2004, http://endeavors.unc.edu/win2004/hugs.html.

Meditate

Research shows benefits, but if it's not for you, don't start here. Remember that we redefined meditation, so you don't have to think of it as sitting with your legs crossed trying not to fall asleep. Listen to relaxing music or a guided meditation, stare at a candle, try to stay focused while you complete a mundane task, color in a coloring book, take a class, paint, or walk. Try the breathing exercises in this book. You don't have to meditate alone, and you can define meditation for yourself.

Laugh

This may be the best tip toward mindfulness (plus, it works your abdominal muscles). Grab your favorite funny movie. If you have been in pain a long time, consider how often you laugh, and create opportunities that will entice amusement. Laughter releases endorphins, natural opioids that act as painkillers. When people laugh, their pain threshold goes up. Laughter is 30 times more likely in social settings, so laugh it up with friends. It might be just what the doctor ordered to alleviate pain.

Look forward

This may seem like the opposite of mindfulness, but sometimes it's easy to get caught in the monotony of life. We need activities and experiences to look forward to. Maybe they make us laugh. Maybe they create a new memory we will never forget. Maybe they are a total flop but become a joke going forward. Try to make sure at least once each week, if not every day, you have something you are eagerly anticipating. This could be a designated phone call with a friend, dinner at your favorite restaurant, a bath, a movie, a Broadway show, a music concert, or a get together with friends for games or drinks. No judgement. Whatever you look forward to is the answer.

In WWI, Lieutenant Colonel Henry Beecher, an anesthesiologist, was in Europe assessing over 200 seriously injured soldiers. When offered morphine, 75 percent declined. Beecher was baffled. Back home, civilians with similar injuries would have pleaded for morphine. The wounded soldiers' lives were about to improve. They were going to return home now, maybe with military honors. On the other hand, civilians in severe pain experienced a sudden drop in quality of life. Simply knowing something good is headed your way can release endorphins that help minimize pain. Like the placebo effect, it's not all in your head. Physical hormones release into your system that make you feel better, so plan for events that you know make you feel good.

CHAPTER 7: COMMON EXERCISE CONCERNS

When we are in pain, we are wise not to risk causing more pain in our body. Let's take a moment to review some common exercise concerns people have and how to adjust for them. Learning to move from the right place is how we keep from creating pain in the body long term by repeating hurtful movement patterns.

How Do I Engage My Abs Without Hurting My Neck or Back?

Very often when exercising (or after exercising) the abdominals, people feel a strain in the neck or back. Repeating the exercise without altering where you feel discomfort can lead to prolonged neck and back pain, and teaches the body that ab work comes with pain, a lesson we don't want imbedded in our minds. Learning to engage and make the abdominal muscles work can be a surprising challenge. Remember, we have more than that dreamy six-pack muscle. The muscles beneath and beside the abdominal muscles are the real answer to reducing back pain, creating fantastic abs, and developing a well-balanced body.

You may have heard a fitness instructor (most likely a Pilates instructor) say "Scoop the abs," "Draw the belly button to the spine," "Zip the jeans," or "Engage the abs." There are endless ways to say it, but only one way to do it. It's subtle and can be a challenge to figure out how to do accurately. Those cues are trying to get you to engage your deepest abdominal muscle, the transversus abdominis (TA). Let's try finding your TA, shall we? This movement is not meant to feel like you are sucking your stomach in until you can't breathe. (You'll notice in the picture that the increments are very subtle.) It should be gentle and feel like it creates a taut feeling from pubic bone to belly button. I cue, "Imagine putting on skinny jeans fresh from the dryer after eating Thanksgiving dinner." But if larger concepts and big visuals help you understand, initially think of being punched in the gut. I hate that cue, but sometimes I find it is easier to rein in a big movement than try to start with a small one.

Movement Break: TA Engagement

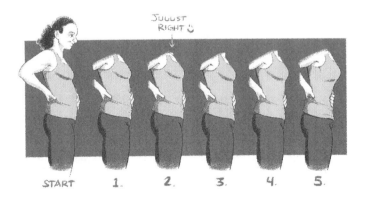

This movement break will take you through how to gently engage your TA. We'll start with big moves (because sometimes that is easier to feel), but in the end, this should be a delicate sensation.

- Find a comfortable position sitting, lying down, or on all fours.

- As you breathe, start by taking a few belly breaths. You'll notice your stomach moves in and out with the breath.

- Then on an exhale, actively engage the abs segmentally five times, pulling the abs in a little deeper, a little deeper, etc.

- Repeat, and notice what you felt when you engaged a little deeper the second time (level two). That is the sweet spot. Remember to shoot for a gentle feeling of skin tautness. Make sure you can still breathe.

- When you inhale, you might lose the connection a little. That is okay. Reconnect on the exhale.

- Repeat for a minute.

- NOTE: You can see in the illustration how subtle this is. It's hard to tell the difference from image to image, but you can see the change from beginning to end. At level two, there should not be an extremely noticeable result.

Be gentle with yourself. (I know I keep saying this, but it's important. In order to heal, you need to be gentle.) Feel the muscle gently wrap around your body. Let this be where your greatest stabilization and your deepest strength comes from.

When people try to engage their abs on command, they often also imprint the spine as if the two things are one and the same. Imprint versus neutral is a reference to positioning the low back and pelvis. *Imprint versus neutral is a different concept from engaging your abs.* People often confuse the two or link the two together. When you do pelvic tilts or rock from imprint to neutral, your pelvis SHOULD move. When you zip the jeans, the pelvis SHOULD NOT move. Sometimes you zip and tuck in combination, but you do not have to. It's important to know that you can engage the abdominals without being imprinted. You do not want to strive to be imprinted all day. But gentle abdominal engagement can help support the low back.

Imprint is when you gently lengthen your low back. If you were lying on the floor, you feel your entire low back against the floor as if you are gently pressing and making an impression of your spine against the ground. Neutral is when you have the natural curve of the lower back in the spine, so there would be a slight arch. The size of that arch differs for everyone. A frequent image used to describe the two positions is to imagine that you have a cup of tea on your lower abs. You are lying on the floor with legs bent, feet on the floor. In neutral that tea is balanced and level in the cup. When you rock to imprint, slightly tucking your tailbone between your legs, the tea spills out of the cup onto your stomach. (See Movement Break: The Pelvic Tilt on page 166)

Whether neutral or imprinted, we should be able to zip, scoop, or engage our abs. When doing ab exercises with our feet on the floor, we should strive to stay neutral. It's the best position since it's the natural position for the spine. We don't want to tuck our tailbone between our legs and lengthen our low back all day long. This position aggravates the back over time. If our low back is lengthened constantly, we remove the natural curve and make every movement more compressive on the spine. A functional TA is vital to a healthy back, because our TA aids in steadying the lumbar spine (low back). We need our abs slightly activated throughout the day when we sit, stand, walk, or run so that they can help stabilize us without force. You can work on this anywhere: the office, on a walk, at a football game, in church, watching TV, cooking dinner. Plus, our abdominals help support all our internal organs. Weak abs that do not provide support allow everything inside us to basically hang off our spine, placing constant pressure on the back.

Another misconception people have is that you have to be lying down to be imprinted. I think this comes from where we most readily use it, lying down in a fitness class. Instructors often cue to press the low back toward the mat. You can imprint in any position (lying on your back, lying on your stomach, on all fours, sitting, or standing). If your lower back lengthens and your pelvis tucks under, you are imprinting the spine. The floor is a helpful place to learn imprint, because having the floor to feel as you move is beneficial to understanding how the movement feels. The floor provides sensation and proprioception.

If you are still not sure you are engaging the TA or can't feel it, try to do a Kegel. When you engage the Kegel (the muscles of the pelvic floor), the TA will automatically fire. Or try standing up straight and pressing your toes into the floor as if you wanted to curl them under but can't because the floor is in the way. Still can't feel it? Keep practicing or playing. It will come. Sometimes it takes time, especially if you've ever had any kind of abdominal surgery (C-section included). Keep playing and exploring. Don't give up. You can do this. Think about it daily at every streetlight, doorknob, text alert, or phone call until it sticks! Once you start to understand how to engage your deep abdominals to support and protect the back in ab exercises, it should help with every task in life.

If it is your neck that bothers you when you do ab exercises, it is more often about positioning. If you have a neck injury (whiplash, a disc-related issue, or slept on it funny), you can relax. That is not pain you want to work through. You may need to rein in the exercises you are doing and only do ab work with the head down for the time being or use props to help you find a more comfortable working position. Don't be deceived; you can get a good abdominal challenge with your head on the floor. I like to refer to different positions as "different" hard rather than declaring one move harder than another, especially since what is harder can be based on body type and an individual's personal strengths and weaknesses. However, if you have your legs in the air for an ab exercise and you choose to keep your head down, it is typically harder to maintain imprint than if you curl your head up. If you keep your head down, your abs are still getting plenty of work.

The body is smart. It will find ways to make an exercise easier. When the neck aches, the abs are being slackers, the school bullies who want the nerdy muscles to do their homework for them. Because your neck is made up of much smaller muscles than the abdominals, the neck cannot do the work of the abs without pain. That's not their role. Or perhaps the reason your neck feels strained during ab exercises is due to faulty alignment, meaning your head is forward, your chin is crammed to your chest, or your head is dangling back in space. Your neck is not in-line with your spine.

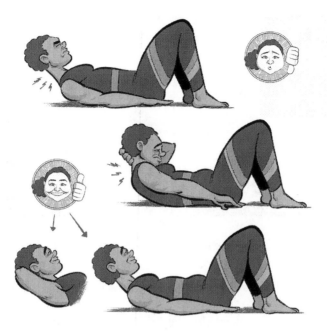

Your hands can be behind your head for a little support (never yanking the head forward) or at your sides hovering off the ground.

Most of the time, if you can play around with the positioning of your head (pull it back in space, tilt it up slightly or down slightly), you can find a place where that pain goes away or at least greatly diminishes. Often, that place will be where you feel more work in the abs. Now that you have fully learned to utilize your abdominals, you may not be able to do as many repetitions. But isn't that the point—finding the right muscle? Take your time and build up to more repetitions. Less is more once you are moving right. It takes time to strengthen and retrain the body. It's better to do two quality movements than ten that cause neck strain and make no change. Listen to your body and allow yourself to build slowly. Our desire for immediate progress forces us into positions that cause pain and may even add to the existing problem. Then we hurt. Then we blame movement. Then we stop moving. Then we hurt worse. It's an endless cycle. We all have the power to end this continuous cycle of pain.

How to Stabilize Without Tension

Whenever we move, we need to retain stability for our safety. You know this intuitively. It's why so many people throw their back out picking up something lightweight like a tissue. When you go to lift a rock, you brace, prepare, and stabilize without thinking. When you go to lift a crumpled paper, you aren't worried, but your back gets thrown out. Even when you lift a feather, there is a lot happening in the body that requires stabilization. The body still needed to tense effectively. Tension becomes a problem when it presents as unnecessary gripping. Think of when you realize your shoulders are shrugged up to your ears when you are cold, holding something heavy, stuck in traffic, or sitting in a frustrating meeting. You need to stabilize without gripping or bearing down, which can be surprisingly complicated.

One of the major principles of Pilates is stability. We stabilize the pelvis and low back before every movement by engaging the deep abdominal muscles first. The reason for this is to protect our bodies from strain and pain. For a while in my personal practice, I took the concept of stability too intensely. I went over the top, persistently concentrating on stabilizing until Pilates became frustrating. It's the type A in me. I was almost moving aggressively, jarring, gripping, and bearing down. Tell me to stabilize, and I want to be the best little stabilizer you've ever seen. Engaging a muscle gently and quietly without cramming or forcing is a unique challenge, at least for me. But I don't think I'm alone. We are an all-or-nothing society. If you are so stable that you become rigid, then you can't move. In Pilates, it is equally important to maintain a flexible, mobile spine. It becomes a fine balance between the stability and mobility, activating a muscle so that it feels like a supportive sling without restricting movement. I'm still working on this concept in my body. Stabilizing and relaxing at the same time sometimes feels impossible. The goal is to stabilize and maintain mobility.

When in pain, simple tasks we once took for granted, like walking, become unbearable. We need to make walking (or any move) look and feel easy again, striving to be simultaneously stable and supple with time, practice, patience, and motivation. Our bodies brace when we are in pain. We tense as a protective mechanism to minimize the pain or preserve our safety. For a sudden injury, bracing is protective, but long-term bracing leads to chronic pain. Bad tension leads to more strain.

The process may be a challenge along the way. There may be setbacks. That's okay. The first step is to notice during your day when you feel rigid. Are your shoulders up to your ears? Is your jaw clenched? Try to relax a little. See how that feels. Do you feel vulnerable? When standing, if I relax my quads in the front of my thighs (which are overdeveloped and tight), I feel like I could topple over and lose my balance. Other times, like when I relax my shoulders or back, I feel at ease by releasing tension in my body. Relaxing different parts of my body creates a different response.

Movement Break: The Pelvic Tilt

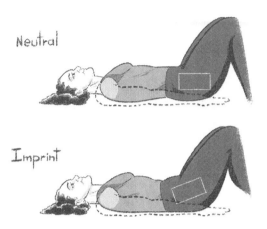

Neutral

Imprint

Every joint in the body has its own neutral. Here, we will go over the pelvis in neutral, but it is not only a term for the lower back. We will be using this movement to explore how you can move without tension, so notice if you can do this movement and feel relaxed at the same time.

- Lie down on your back, knees bent and feet on the floor. Arms relaxed at your sides.

- Rock your pelvis from neutral (slight arch in the low back) to imprint (spine lengthening toward the floor without being forceful).

- Observe what you feel. Do you feel tension? Are you cramming anything? Are you squeezing your butt? Are other parts of your body moving (your head, your shoulders, your ribs, your legs)? Does it feel like the movement happens naturally, or you jam your bones in one direction or the other?

If you said yes to any of these, you might want to practice easing into your stabilization and using less force. Be gentle with yourself. If you do feel tension, how do you let that tension go but still hold a position in the body? Start by making adjustments to the points you noticed above. Are you squeezing your butt? Relax your glutes without changing where your pelvis is. Hopefully, that creates a little relief. Try making the movement smaller, even if it feels like you are barely moving. Make it so small that nothing else moves. Play with that until it becomes second nature and feels easy. Then you can play with increasing the movement, but it's never going to be huge. Stability comes from small adjustments. Our stabilizer muscles are not our major movers.

Remind yourself during workouts that when you are trying to hone your stabilization skills, sometimes less is more. For instance, if you do any exercise on your back with your legs in the air, you may notice your shoulders are tense. To relax them, you may have to make whatever movement you are doing smaller. For most of us, doing exercises properly usually means less range of motion. People get turned off, because they want big moves. But the little move works you harder and yields more results. You must alter your mindset. If your shoulders tense, your abs are straining and searching for other muscles to get involved and reduce the abdominals' workload. Build slowly. If you force yourself to a position you can't stabilize yet, you will wind up in pain over time. Sync the movement to your breathing. Use your exhale as the reminder to gently engage. If you lose the connection a little on the inhale, that is normal and okay. Reconnect on the exhale.

If this all sounds overwhelming, once in a while, as long as you are in a safe position, just let the body move freely. That, too, is part of the learning.

Things to Consider Before You Start Moving

Daniel Wolpert is a neuroscientist and engineer who argues that the reason we have evolved with brains is to move. I fell in love with him almost immediately. He explains that the sea squirt (a potato-shaped invertebrate that lives in the sea) has a central nervous system and moves around in the water. Eventually, the filter-feeding sea squirt finds a place with a satisfying amount of food and a pleasing temperature, at which point it settles down for a life forever attached to a rock and then consumes its own brain. If it helps you deal with some of your pain, maybe this is a reminder that you should never get too comfortable. Being uncomfortable encourages us to strive for a better life and motivates us to move.

If you are happy to have a brain, it's time to move your body. The collection of exercises in the next section was created to reduce pain throughout your body. You don't have to limit yourself to these movements, but try them all. Star the ones that feel particularly good. Everything you've been practicing and learning thus far should be incorporated into these movements. Pick which actions are best for your body based on your needs. It won't all come at once. That's okay. Practice makes progress.

We tend to believe that someone (our doctor, physical therapist, personal trainer) can tell us what exercises to do. Experts do have an understanding of the body and injuries and should be able to guide you. Still, no one knows your body as well as you. Never forget that. You need a dialogue with your healthcare provider or exercise therapist. If you have found relief using standard exercises that work for most people, it's less of an issue. But if you feel stuck and everything you have tried hasn't worked, you need to talk to them about what you're really experiencing in your body. Tell them what feels good or bad, what exhausts you or provides an energy boost. The better you can relay that to a practitioner you are working with, the better they will be able to advise you. Also, be okay telling someone, "No. I am not comfortable doing that. I don't think it helps because it hurts." Having someone you trust and can dialogue with makes a difference.

I am endlessly baffled by clients, friends, and family who go to a practitioner and work through extreme pain. Not that it couldn't or wouldn't happen, but I have never seen anyone I know improve through this process. Pain begets pain. You must learn to move without pain or you train the body to move with it. In 2011, a small study interviewed patients and providers about how they felt about Pain Induced by Exercise and Mobilization (PIEM). Patients were either ambivalent or felt negatively toward PIEM. Providers more often emphasized the positive aspects of PIEM. While practitioners believed PEIM had positive effects, it resulted in worse conditions, fears, and rejection toward physical therapy and did not prevent or reduce stress patients felt about pain. The study concluded that there should be better communication among everyone involved.[54] I know so much more about the body and movement than most of my clients. Still, if one of them tells me they feel something happening in their body, good or bad, even if it is not what I expected or intended, they are always right. We can discuss it, but what they feel is more important than what I see or expect to be true. If I can teach them to trust what they feel, I am doing them a service. We need to see practitioners as facilitators, not necessarily healers. It's a team effort. There is no magic, and good communication will help.

Please don't be mistaken here. I'm not saying physical therapy is bad or that you should be scared to go. There are wonderful

---

54 Sophie Alami et al., "Management of Pain Induced by Exercise and Mobilization during Physical Therapy Programs: Views of Patients and Care Providers," *BMC Musculoskeletal Disorders* 12 (2011): 172, https://doi.org/10.1186/1471-2474-12-172.

physical therapists doing great work, and people should probably be sent to physical therapy more often than they currently are. But dialogue with them, and if they aren't willing to engage in conversation and work you without pain, seek another practitioner. At the very least, make them explain their reasoning and provide research. If someone is intimidated by you asking them to explain themselves, they don't have much confidence in what they do, especially since research is showing that explanation helps relieve pain. We are more motivated to do something if we can rationalize how it will help us. Adults are more apt to accept new information if it is relevant to them and solves a problem. This is a crucial factor in adult learning theory.

Chronic pain develops over time, and it will take focus and retraining to undo. You are charting a new course, embarking on an adventure to discover healing sensations throughout your body. Experiment and explore. If it hurts, stop. Continue with what feels good. Trust your body. It will tell you what it does and does not like. Trust your body's sense of self-preservation. If you switch your mindset to observing your body as it moves, your body will develop more control. You'll start to notice pain as it approaches, so you can stop and try another course. When building a habit or lifelong routine, seek pleasure. Try all the exercises in this book. Do the ones that challenge you. Do the ones that feel good. Skip the ones that aggravate something or feel dreadful. Go back now and again and try something you once hated. As the body changes, you might find a new favorite exercise.

The next section of this book includes exercises that generally only require your body. A pillow or yoga mat may increase comfort. When a half foam roller is used, a thicker book, like a dictionary, or a rolled-up yoga mat can be substituted. A medium weight flex band is optional.

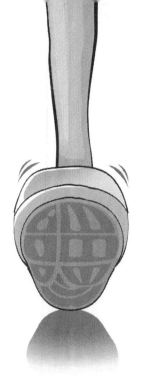

SECTION THREE:
THE MOVES

"If something stands between you and your success, move it. Never be denied."

—Dwayne "The Rock" Johnson

It's officially time to get moving. The next chapters will break movements up into parts of the body: Happy Feet, Happy Hips & Low Back, and Happy Neck & Shoulders. If you have a specific injury and want to skip ahead to a specific part, that is okay, but remember every part of the body is interconnected. The first exercise in Happy Feet is likely beneficial for most people. If you skip ahead for now, come back and try everything later. You might be surprised what helps. Sometimes backing off the area in pain and working something else frees you up to do movements you are less worried about and reminds you that you can still move. Each section will provide some information about that area of your body and will then list a few helpful exercises.

CHAPTER 8: HAPPY FEET

Before we explore our feet too much, let's get a baseline for how they feel.

Movement Break: Feel Your Feet

Walk around the room barefoot (if you can safely) and answer these questions:

What do you notice about your feet?

Do you walk heel-toe, or do you land on the ball of your foot?

Can you tell if you walk on the outside or inside of your foot?

Are your feet angled in (pigeon-toed) or out (duck-footed)?

Do your feet feel good, bad, indifferent, sensitive, nothing?

Does the surface you are on (wood, carpet, tile) seem to matter?

There are no wrong answers. If your current answer is "I don't know," that is okay.

Your Feet!

Our feet have 26 bones, take about 8,000 steps a day, and support one million pounds of pressure in an hour-long walk. Our feet bear the burden of our weight and movement each day, yet we don't often pay much attention to our feet. The happier our feet are, the stronger, more efficient, and more functional our body is. Perhaps we should give our tenacious tootsies a little more consideration. If you have knee, hip, or back pain, your feet may be an important component of that issue. These exercises will bring you in touch with your sole. We'll work on arch strength; toe, foot, and ankle mobility and flexibility; bunion and hammertoe care; plantar fasciitis release; and balance. Want to get the spring back in your step? Keep reading.

We are pretty tough on our feet and often take them for granted. According to a Pilates elder I trained with, if someone went to Joseph Pilates for a back injury, he would often spend 30 minutes exercising their feet. He believed that if the feet weren't right, nothing else would feel right. You have to work the body as a whole, but starting with your feet is like working the border of a puzzle; it's a manageable place to start solving the whole mystery. If the feet are not in good condition, that problem creeps up the rest of your body and affects everything else. If you roll in on your feet (fallen arches or *pronating*) or roll out (high arches or *supinating*), that is going to affect your knees, hips, and back.

Footwear

Part of your morning ritual probably includes donning a pair of shoes. At least 40,000 years ago, we started shoving our feet into shoes. Some anthropologists believe our toes have gotten shorter because of shoes.[55] Others think wimpy toes came from diminished movement when we wear shoes. Either way, the way shoes restrict our feet means what we put on for fashion or protection deserves some consideration.

Shoes were not created to harm us, and while they serve as a protective mechanism when walking on sidewalks that might be littered with gravel and broken glass, it is possible for shoes to do damage. Shoes change the shape and structure of your frame. When you wear high heels or shoes with a positive heel lift (the case with almost every shoe, including men's shoes and sneakers), you shorten your calf muscles and alter the stiffness and thickness of the Achilles tendon.[56] A positive heel means that the heel is higher than the ball of your foot. Even a slight heel lift can alter your body. This change in musculature can result in and exacerbate knee pain, back pain, and migraines. The feet affect body parts all the way up to your head.

Armed with knowledge of footwear and foot anatomy, you can evaluate the shoes you wear most often. Here's what's best:

Your heel should be negative or flat. A minimal postive heel is not the end of the world, but when the heel is one inch or higher, we shift our weight and place strain on areas not well-equiped for it. Heels increase the weight and pressure on the forefoot. Toes need space, so the toe box should be big and allow the toes to

---

55 Maggie Koerth-Baker, "First Shoes Worn 40,000 Years Ago," *Live Science*. Purch, June 5, 2008.
56 Meagen Voss, "Why High Heels Hurt Even After You Take Them Off." *NPR*, July 15, 2010.

move freely. Most of our shoes fit snugly around our toes or crush our toes together, which is linked to bunions. The sole should be thin and flexible. If it's not thin, look for flexible. If it's too rigid or thick, the shoe will limit sensation to the nerves of the foot and reduce mobility of the muscles in the foot and lower leg. A fully flexible shoe should be twistable like when you wring out a towel. The shoe should be well-attached, meaning a flip-flop (which I admit to wearing daily) is not as good for our feet as a sandal with a strap that holds itself on. With flip-flops, toes have to grip in an unnatural way to hold the flip-flop on. It may be a contributing factor to developing hammertoe.

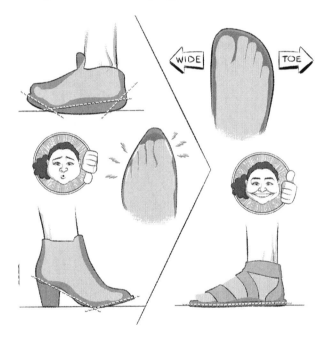

Arch support is a sticky one. Lots of people with flat feet think they need it, and we all are trained to believe we need it. It can help reduce pain, but it doesn't resolve the problem. If everything is functioning properly with our foot, we shouldn't require arch support. The sole of our foot has multiple arches, but usually arch support is there for the medial arch, the one we are most familiar with and can picture under the inside edge of the foot. Our anatomy is pretty spectacular. That arch, like the arch of a bridge, is structurally designed to support our body. It would seem preposterous to constantly jam something up against the keystone or center of an arch of a bridge. We know doing so would ultimately weaken the structure of the bridge if we regularly applied pressure against it from beneath. Yet that is exactly what arch support like orthotics do to our foot; it's conceptually a good idea but potentially injurious in daily practice. Constantly pushing up on the structure weakens the foot. The body is smart (or lazy) and takes the path of least resistance. Provide something for the arch to rest upon and the muscles will weaken and let the fabricated support system do the work. Orthotics alone are not the enemy. They can alleviate pain for some people almost immediately, making them a brilliant creation. However, if you are using orthotics, it becomes even more vital that you do foot exercises. Think of orthotics like a neck brace. You would never be content if your doctor told you that you had to spend the rest of your life in a neck brace; you shouldn't be happy to hear that you have to spend the rest of your life in orthotics. They are the same fix: a Band-Aid, not a lifelong solution. Shoes can come with support that weakens our feet over time. We didn't evolve to need a cobbler. It's not that you shouldn't wear shoes or orthotics, but the more you wear them, the more you need to exercise and rebuild your feet.

Shoes are practical and fashionable. I have no intention of giving up shoes. But recognize that footwear limits the range of motion your foot is supposed to have. Footwear generally confines us to pointing and flexing at the ankle. The muscles of the lower leg and foot are meant to do so much more than that. They can roll the foot from side to side. Your foot can have the same mobility and dexterity as your dominant hand. In a pinch, and with training, your feet can act as hands minus opposable thumbs. In shoes, your feet deteriorate. But it's not hopeless.

If you go shopping for better shoes, keep in mind that a sudden change can be harmful. High-heel wearers often complain about how their feet hurt when walking barefoot. Walking barefoot is exactly what they need, but most of us can't handle going cold turkey. Spending five to ten minutes a day barefoot or in flats could be plenty for someone who is used to a high heel. Progress slowly. Start with slightly lower heels. If you don't have any intention of changing your footwear, spend a few minutes a day without shoes and do these exercises. It's not all or nothing. You can think like an urbanite: heels at work, pumps during the commute, and slippers or barefoot before bed. Gradual changes and variety is best.

It's not just the heel lift, squished toes, and arch that create a problem for our feet. The actual padding does us harm in the long run. A 1997 study at McGill University found that runners land harder the more padding they have on the foot.[57] Padding was intended to absorb shock, but when we wear padding we have a harder foot strike, potentially creating more shock. The theory: our feet need to feel the ground to balance. If padding blocks the sensation, the body tries harder to feel. Without sensation, the body can't tell where it is in space. The same was found of gymnasts landing on firmer surfaces.[58]   Meant to provide support and protection, shoes have actually left our feet desperately in search of sensation and stability. Feeling is how the body senses itself in space. It wants to feel. Allow it a few minutes of bare feeling every day.

Kick off your clogs and move or walk barefoot in a safe location where debris can't hurt you, like inside your home or in a plot

---

57 Adam Sternbergh, "You Walk Wrong," *New York Magazine*, April 21, 2008.
58 Sternbergh, "You Walk Wrong."

of lush grass. It's good for the musculature of your foot that becomes weak and lethargic in shoes. Walking barefoot benefits the nervous system and improves balance. If the practice causes pain, stop. Creating more or different pain is contrary to your overall good.

Minimalist Footwear

A few years ago, minimalist footwear was all the rage, especially for runners. Its bad reputation blossomed when many injuries were associated with the unsupportive footwear. The likely problem: most people switched footwear suddenly without transitioning slowly.[59] Even if you are in great shape, your body becomes accustomed to the life you've been giving it. One of my friends was a runner who transferred to sneakers without support. Many minimalist footwear websites suggested progressing slowly and starting with as little as half a mile if you had previously spent a lifetime running in regular sneakers. Very few converts, especially runners, had the willpower to wait. Many went about their normal runs of six miles or more suddenly expecting tendons and muscles that had not engaged in years to operate effectively. My friend injured both of his Achilles tendons. Many people in the same boat blamed the footwear. It wasn't the footwear. Their bodies were not prepared for the footwear, and they needed to start slowly. Our body requires time to retrain the muscles of the lower leg and foot.

In theory, minimalist footwear should be better for all our activities, from running, walking, or playing certain sports. They should protect our feet from debris and rough surfaces (although stubbing your toe while hiking in minimalist footwear is no fun), and they encourage and enable more movement of the foot and

---

59 Kathryn Doyle, "Switch to Minimalist Running Shoes Tied to Injuries, Pain," *Reuters*, January 9, 2014.

lower leg. In sneakers (which I wear and am not against), the foot cannot move much. It allows for movement at the ankle, but toe movement is restricted and often curled upward. We are meant to have movement of the forefoot called *inversion* and *eversion* (movements that tilt the sole of the foot toward or away from the body). In shoes that offer us a lot of support, that movement is restricted so the muscles work less and become unprepared to support and balance our body, weight, and movement.

Part Nature, Part Nurture

For most of my life, it was presumed that foot problems like bunions were genetic, and therefore we were doomed to get them if Grandma had them. Now, it is presumed multiple circumstances might result in a bunion. In addition to genetics, footwear plays an important role. Perhaps most interestingly, learning to walk and move from someone who has a bunion (like our mom or grandma) possibly also increases our chances of getting that painful outcropping of bone at our big toe. When we copy their walking pattern, we copy the type of movement that would lead to a bunion. The good news is that if we can learn a behavior, we can unlearn it. Exercises and proper movements are crucial for resolving painful patterns. Once a bunion or hammertoe exists, it's harder to correct. Catch a problem before there is pain, and you'll be better off long term.

Bunion: a painful, bony bump on the first joint of the big toe. You can often see that the angle of the big toe changes, pushing into the rest of the toes.

Hammertoe: a toe that is bent downward, usually as a result of pressure from footwear. It looks like the joint in the toe sticks up.

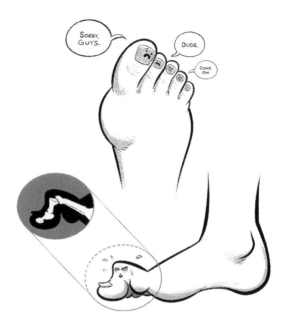

These foot problems can be exacerbated by our daily movement. Simply walking can increase the problem or the discomfort. When we walk, our gait is intended to have our legs parallel. But if someone has a lateral turn out (think duck feet) and then they pronate (think fallen arches or flat feet) as they walk, their body weight puts more pressure on that big toe joint with every step. That might cause a bunion to develop, and it certainly might aggravate an existing bunion more. But we are capable of altering our gait pattern. Next time you go for a walk, for part of that walk, notice which directions your toes point. Notice what muscles you feel working the most, where you put pressure in your foot, and how or if you roll through your foot. Simply start to notice. It's the first step in making a change. You can play with different leg and foot positions for a short time and see how they feel differently to your body while you are walking. Notice how you feel after the walk if you've made any changes. But remember, start with a few moments of change.

The Ankle Joint

The very mobile ankle has to bear all our weight all day. Generally, we want and need to maintain ankle mobility. For the health of your ankle, consider many of the exercises in this segment. You might find it fun or helpful to go to a shoe store or doctor and have your ankles assessed. Do you pronate (roll in flattening your arch), supinate (roll out with a high arch), or have a neutral ankle? You may already know the answer by looking at a pair of shoes. Do you wear away the inside edge (most likely a pronator) or do you wear away the outside edge (supinator) more quickly? Find out what group you fall in, and do exercises to strengthen the lower leg muscles to help create a more neutral ankle. It's vital to strengthen your ankle, because a weak ankle will trickle up to every part of your body.

The Fascia You Have Heard Of: Plantar Fascia

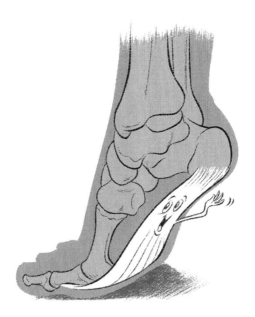

One of the more common problems with the feet is *plantar fasciitis*. Remember your new friend fascia?   Plantar fascia is typically the only way most people have heard of it. Plantar fasciitis—one of the most common causes of heel pain—involves discomfort and inflammation on the thick band of tissue that runs across the bottom of your foot and connects your heel to your toes. It provides support for the arch of the foot. The plantar fascia also plays a dynamic role in gait. With each step as we roll off the toes, the plantar fascia shortens, making the foot more rigid. When we land, the plantar fascia is lengthened, allowing for suppleness in the foot.

That painful band of fascia in your sole ultimately connects to the whole body, transforming into your Achilles tendon, intertwining around everything up the back of your body, and reaching the brow of your forehead as it encapsulates various muscles. The fascia is playing that endless game of tug-of-war. Something always has to give. If the plantar fascia is inflamed because the calf is tight, the hamstrings may have to loosen, the glute may have to tighten, the back lengthens, the shoulders tighten, the neck loosens, and the back of the skull to the crown of the head tightens. Whether loose or tight, an area can experience pain. Think of pain or discomfort moving through the body with a whip effect. A small change in the lower part of your body grows as it moves up. When you snap a whip, you produce a small motion with your wrist, but the end farther from your hand sustains a sizeable movement. Likewise, if something is out of alignment at your feet that alters your natural movement, a large shift happens at your neck and head.

The Exercises

As you do the following exercises, try them on different surfaces. Remember, even if you can't tell the difference, your nervous system denotes variance, and your nervous system wants variety. The soles of our feet have over 200,000 nerve endings, one of the most nerve-populated areas of our body. Our feet are created to guide us with constant feedback, serving as a probe between us and the world. But we shield them and ultimately shield ourselves from feeling. As we age, our nervous system changes and experiences the world around us differently. While we tend to have an increase in pain as we get older, we tend to physically feel less. This is potentially one of the reasons seniors are more prone to falls; they can't feel where they are in space as well as they once used to. Exercise and movement are vital for healthy longevity. Instead of becoming afraid to move, we must move. Moving strengthens the muscles so that they can compensate for the changes in sensation.

Let's jump into the exercises feet first!

These exercises will start to wake your feet up. Waking up any body part we haven't paid attention to can help change holding patterns in other parts of our body that have become locked as well. Maybe you feel stuck somewhere else. Move your feet for a bit. Wiggle your toes. No movement is wasted. Do not feel limited to the exercises below. Some may not work for you initially, but others will feel fantastic from the first try. Remember, always cycle back. Try the ones you didn't fall madly in love with at first glance.

Consider rubbing your feet an exercise. Rub each foot for two-and-a-half minutes when you get in bed. Or get a racket ball and use it to rub your foot, rolling it around or gently pressing down on the ball. Never press or apply pressure that hurts. Pain is not our goal. Reduced pain is the goal. Play: you don't need a special technique to stimulate the nervous system as far as anyone knows. Do what feels good and remember creativity is welcome when you move.

You'll see the first exercise repeated in the section on Happy Hips & Low Back. That is how important it is.

> Real people posed for these illustrations. You'll find some of my clients, family, and friends who were instrumental in the making of this book!

Calf Stretch.

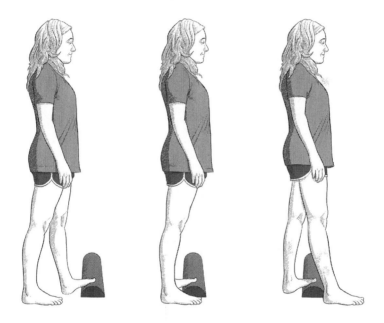

Place the ball of your foot on top of the half foam roller or rolled-up yoga mat, heel on floor, foot straight. Weight should stay in the heels, including the foot on the dome. As if taking one step forward, place the other foot (off to the side of the roller) hip distance apart. Make sure this foot is also straight. Breathe and hold for 15 to 30 seconds. Repeat with the opposite foot. Repeat both feet up to three times. NOTE: When you first attempt this stretch, you are unlikely to have enough calf flexibility to take a full step forward. It is okay if your foot is even with (or behind) the stretching foot at first. It is more important that you keep the weight on the heel of the stretching leg, upper body vertical (if you are really tight, you may try to compensate by leaning forward), and hips square.

Calf Stretch Bent Knee. Set up for the Calf Stretch above. From your stretch position (or with the floor leg a little farther back), slightly bend and straighten both legs. It is a small move. You can hold with a bent leg for 15 to 30 seconds or keep bending and straightening. Repeat up to three times each side.

Toe Lift Series. Standing upright with both feet on the floor, legs hip distance apart, toes pointing forward. Keep the ball of the foot down and only lift the toes without shifting your weight backwards.

Toe Lifts. Lift all 10 toes off the ground. Try to lift the pinkie toes as much as the big toes. Hold for a couple breaths, then lift and lower toes rhythmically eight to ten times. *Add a toe spread:* Lift toes, spread the toes as wide as possible, then lay foot down. Repeat eight to ten times.

Big Toe Lifts. Begin holding all 10 toes off ground. Try to put both big toes down on floor. Hold it there for a few seconds. When you've mastered that challenge, begin to tap and release big toes.

Pinkie Toe Lifts. Same thing on the other end. Begin holding all 10 toes off the ground. Try to place down the pinkie toes while holding all eight other toes off mat. Once you master that movement, tap repeatedly.

Alternating Toe Lifts. Now try to alternate taps between the big toes and the pinkie toes. Keep repeating for about 30 to 45 seconds. At end of challenge, try to put big toes and pinkie toes down at the same time while holding the three center toes off the ground. If you cannot do this right away, don't worry.

Point & Flex. Sitting or lying on your back with the legs in the air (you can hold your legs with your hands for support), point and flex the foot.

Slow Point & Flex.

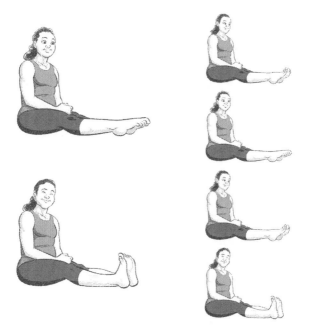

Sitting or lying on your back with the legs in the air, point and flex the foot. But break it down. First push through the ball of your foot (looks like you have Barbie feet), then point the toes. Then to return, pull your toes back and then flex the foot at the ankle.

Circles. Sitting or lying on your back with the legs in the air (you can hold your legs with your hands), circle the ankles in each direction.

Pronate and Supinate/Eversion and Inversion.

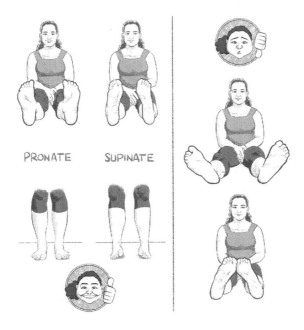

PRONATE   SUPINATE

Sit with legs straight. Without letting your whole leg move and trying to keep the movement at the ankle, move your feet from left to right as if the bottoms of the feet want to look at each other and then they turn away from each other. Sometimes this movement is easier to find when standing.

CHAPTER 9: HAPPY HIPS & LOW BACK

Our pelvis supports 80 bones in our upper body and transfers some of that weight to our legs. The pelvis and back are intertwined. You cannot move one without the other, so if your pelvis is tilted or crooked, your back is too. It can be a heavy burden to bear for the hip joint and the lumbar vertebrae, especially when we have poor posture. The second most common joint replacement surgery is a hip replacement (trailing behind knee surgery, which can be due to an original hip issue). According to the Centers for Disease Control, hip replacements are on the rise, more than doubling from 2000 to 2010 when they totaled 310,800 in people over 45.[60] This chapter provides exercises to keep your hips and back healthy, so you can enjoy life doing your favorite activities.

---

60 Monica Wolford et al., "Hospitalization for Total Hip Replacement Among Inpatients Aged 45 and Over: United States, 2000–2010," NCHS Date Brief No. 186, February 2015, https://www.cdc.gov/nchs/products/databriefs/db186.htm.

Hydrate for a healthy low back. It's easier to stay hydrated than to play catch up, so grab a glass of water while you read.

Hip and low back pain are linked because of how interconnected the two parts are. The pelvis is the center of the body. Your sacroiliac joints (SI joints for short), those dimples (nicknamed the Dimples of Venus) at the top of your buttock/low back, transfer all the weight up and down the body all day long. Their subtle movement may explain why we underappreciate them as a joint. When listing off the joints of the body (as you do), most people skip right over them.

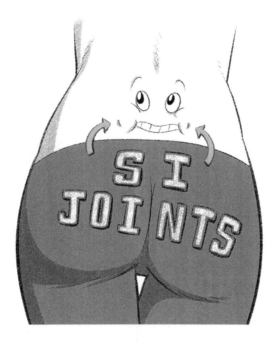

While the pelvis is solid and stable, the lower back is not. Our lower back (lumbar) only has five vertebrae, so it cannot move as much as the neck (which has seven) or mid-back (the thoracic with twelve). Still, when compared to the stability of the pelvis, the lumbar is far more pliable. The lumbar spine twists minimally and bends forward, back, and side to side. The lower vertebrae provide a broad range of motion for which the lumbar spine forfeits stability. Luckily, the body comes with tools to protect and stabilize the lumbar region. Muscles and fascia may be the cause or a complicating factor of your pain right now.

We discussed the transversus abdominis when we learned how to "zip the jeans." The TA protects the spine and maintains a safeguard during movement. Every time you move, whether you are going for a run, picking up a laundry basket, sneezing, or twisting to grab something in the back of your car, three muscles engage milliseconds before movement to protect and stabilize the spine: your TA, your multifidi (small muscles that connect each vertebra in your spine), and the muscles of your pelvic floor (those Kegels). We don't know why, but chronic pain sufferers lose the natural support of the TA. After a back injury, the multifidi become neurologically impaired. If pain is sustained, they atrophy and are replaced with fat.[61] Learning to automatically engage the pelvic floor and TA before movement helps brace and protect our spine, especially important if our muscles may have stopped doing that automatically. As simple as it seems, one of the best things we can do in order to sustain enduring back health is learn to "zip the jeans" and consciously create our own support system before all movement.

Engagement of the TA directly affects the support structure of the lower lumbar spine and the lumbar fascia.

---

61 Michael D. Freedman et al., "The Role of the Lumbar Multifidus in Chronic Low Back Pain: A Review," *PM&R* 2, no. 2 (Feb 2010): 142-46, https://doi.org/10.1016/j.pmrj.2009.11.006.

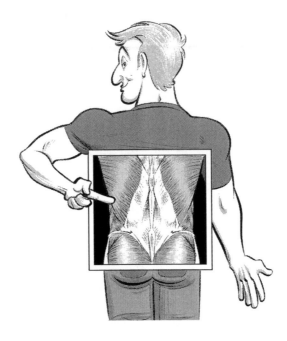

Our lower back has a lot of thick fascia in it. That white stuff is all fascia. Keeping hydrated is so important, because stiff, depleted fascia can restrict movement and create pain. Fascia needs water throughout the day to stay supple in order to operate at peak performance. More often than not, when we pull our back, it isn't simply from the specific incident that brought us to our knees. Most damage to the body is progressive from years of actions that wear down the injured area. Whatever it was that finally did the trick was the straw that broke the camel's back.

Hopefully, you are gently zipping your jeans right now to engage the TA as we move on to the psoas muscle, which we discussed earlier when we were highlighting all the muscles you probably want to know. Your psoas may help flex the hip, but it definitely acts as a spinal stabilizer that connects high on your femur in your thigh and runs over the top of your pelvis where it connects to all your lumbar vertebrae. The poor, exhausted, underappreciated psoas causes a great deal of angst, especially if you spend most of your day sitting. We are a society of tight, weak psoas. Like every muscle in the body, the psoas can be tight or short at one end and weak or long at another. In many bodies, it is pulling the lower back and lower ribs forward in space. While it is meant to support the spine, due to poor posture, it basically yanks on the spine all day long. Letting the psoas rest and achieve a feeling of ease can benefit your back.

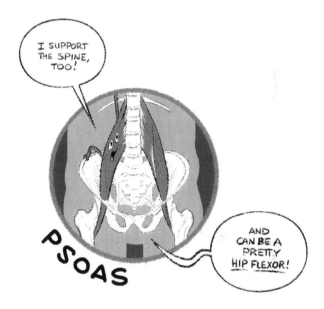

Micro-Movement Break! Constructive Rest

Here's a movement break that actually doesn't require any movement. That's right! You don't need to move to complete this movement break successfully, but it's a wonderful position for your psoas.

- Lie down on a firm surface. A bed will work if getting down on the floor isn't an option, but firmer is better.

- Bend your knees, feet on the floor hip distance apart.

- That's it. Lie there. Breathe.

You are legitimately benefitting your low-back by letting the psoas chill out for a bit. The longer you stay the better, but whatever time you have will do.

You may have heard of your *piriformis* if you've ever had piriformis syndrome or sciatica. The piriformis lives inside your glute. It's deep in your butt beneath the surface. It can cause aggravation when it is too tight. The sciatica nerve runs next to the piriformis, if not imbedded in it. Either way, if the muscle is overly taut, it can put pressure on the nerve creating painful symptoms. If you are ever diagnosed with sciatica, it is important to know whether it originates from something going on in your back or something going on in your butt. Different exercises will provide relief in different scenarios. Ask your doctor.

One of my favorite muscles, the *glute medius*, is located on the side of your pelvis. Have you ever seen an old man shuffle across the room instead of step one foot in front of the other? He needs to shuffle, because he has lost the strength in his glute medius and can no longer balance on one foot for the brief second we have a foot in the air when walking. For long-term mobility and health, you'll want to work your glute medius. Keep in mind that sexy sway women employ when sauntering across a room is a sign of a weak glute medius. High heels can force you into a sexy sway and create a sad, tired glute medius—a red flag for a future hip replacement.

The glute medius may be my favorite in the gluteal range, but all your buttock muscles are important, including the minimus and the maximus. They are directly linked with low back pain. If your glute medius and minimus are not strong and you have that sexy sway, it's not just your hips swaying, the low back is affected with each step. And the glute max enables us to stand upright and erect. It's the largest muscle in the body.

Movement Break: The Flamingo

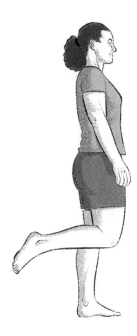

The glute medius assists in balance when you walk. Let's learn which of your glute medius muscles is stronger. People tend to have a more dominant leg that is easier to balance on.

- Doing this exercise barefoot will increase the challenge, but sneakers are an option if that is better for your body.

- Bend one leg back like a flamingo.

- Stand on the other leg, keeping the leg straight but without locking the knee. You should have a soft bend in the floor knee. If you are struggling, place your hand on the wall, using it as much or as little as you need to.

- Try to build up to 60 seconds

- Repeat on the other side.

- Note which side felt easier to balance on.

Gluteal Atrophy or "Oh My Aching Butt!"

Our butts are dying. As a society of sitters, it is no surprise that our butts have begun to atrophy; the largest muscle in our body is literally wasting away. People spend so much time at desks and in cars that our glutes are stretched for upwards of eight hours a day or more. The glutes enable upright, standing posture. They activate when we walk, or at least they should. Our gluteal muscles are our hip extensors, opening up the front of the hip joint. We take this for granted because we are so used to being upright that when we try to extend the hip more from a standing position, we want that movement to be big. The glutes already have extended our hip nearly entirely to get us upright. If we want more hip extension, the glutes can only pull the leg back a little bit farther. If we go too far, we start to overuse our back. Weak glutes or glutes that don't really know when or how to fire are synonymous with back pain.

If any of our glutes are weak, our back will have less stability during movement and even standing. Remember those superficial muscles, the brawny guys we equated to the football jocks. Our glute maximus is the jock that propels us forward and helps us stand up, but unfortunately due to atrophy, our glute max is basically stoned. Women who suffer from chronic low back pain tend to have smaller glute max muscles.[62] The

---

62 Amy H. Amabile et al., "Atrophy of Gluteus Maximus Among Women with a History of Chronic Low Back Pain," *PLOS ONE* 12, no. 7 (2017), https://doi.org/10.1371/journal.pone.0177008.

tired, weak, exhausted glutes peter out faster than their pain-free friend's buttocks. So, like the TA, when we need those muscles the most, they are weary. Proper training becomes key. As you do the exercises in this chapter, check in to ensure you feel your butt firing.

There are two different problems: one with the glute max in the back, the other with the glute medius on the side. Dead butt syndrome is about the glute max, the largest muscle in the body. It's so used to being stretched when we sit and our hip flexors have grown so short and overworked that when we stand up and walk or run, our body falls into what it is used to. The butt doesn't fire to propel us forward, and the hip flexors drag us along. It's great that the body can accommodate our needs, but it doesn't feel good operating this way. The back starts to hurt because muscles of the lower back try to override the glute and do the work or because the psoas yanks on the lower back with each step.

When the glute medius is weak or tired, we tend to hike one hip higher than the other.

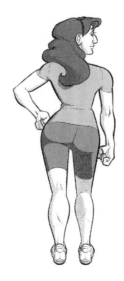

This can happen during every step we take. Think of that sexy hip sway again. Instead of noticing the sexy hips, think of how much unnecessary movement that is placing on the lower back. When your hips move side to side, so does your spine. You want a loose, mobile lumbar spine, but you want it stable when walking, dancing, running, or any activity that requires movement from one foot to the other. Not having the strength in the glute medius to stabilize the pelvis hurts not only the hip joint but also the lower back.

There are quick and easy movements you can do to reverse the decline. Engage your butt whenever you think of it (unless you have sciatica and glute engagement aggravates it). Make sure that doesn't mean tucking your tailbone between your legs. Just like you can engage your abs without moving the position of your pelvis, you can engage your glute max without moving the pelvis. Engage it in the office, in the car, or at the supermarket waiting in line. Try squeezing one side of your butt and then the other, which can help prevent tailbone tucking. Envision a young Arnold Schwarzenegger alternatingly bouncing his pec (chest) muscles up and down. Imagine your glutes lifting like Schwarzenegger's chest muscles. Take your time figuring it out and make it playful. Rome wasn't built in a day, and your butt most likely won't restore itself to *Statue of David* firmness immediately either.

Next time you go for a walk, consider your butt. Do you feel it on every step? No? Play with what you can change in your stride to feel your butt get involved in this very common movement. Try taking a larger stride to see if that helps. Not only will the walking be perking up your butt, but exploring new movement patterns will increase overall muscle tone to parts that may be getting left out.

Movement Break: Squats

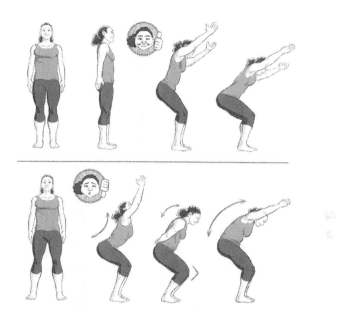

- Stand with your legs hip distance apart, legs parallel, toes pointing forward, *weight over heels.*

- Inhale.

   o Bend your knees as you break at the hips and stick the butt out behind you (like you are looking for a toilet bowl in the dark).

   o As you lower the body, raise the arms to chest height. Your torso should naturally tilt forward a little. Pelvis remains neutral the whole time, torso straight.

   o Stick your tailbone out behind you.

- Exhale.

  o Press the heels into the floor and straighten the legs and hips back up to standing tall.

  o Imagine pushing the floor away with your heels as you straighten your legs. Think of activating your rear, but make sure not to push the pelvis forward at the top.

  o Lower arms to sides.

- Check what you feel: your glutes and legs working, not your back. Throughout the movement, you should be able to lift all 10 toes off the floor. If you cannot, you have too much weight shifted forward. Check your knees. In a squat, your weight should shift back as you lower yourself. Make sure your knees never come forward of your toes. If the knees hurt, start with a smaller range of motion (a partial squat). Keeping the toes lifted should help put less pressure on the knees.

- Repeat up to 12 times. Build up slowly if needed.

The Trouble With Sitting

We sit a lot. It is estimated that we sit on average between nine to ten hours a day. That's 136 days per year of sitting; more than a third of our year is spent in a chair. A few years ago, there was a stream of articles claiming sitting was the new smoking and if you sat down you would die. That is a slight exaggeration, but sitting does create a lot of our aches and pains. Part of the problem stems from the fact that ergonomic chairs aren't actually ergonomic. If your seat has a little bucket seat carved out for your fanny (my Grandma's term), which it probably does, you cannot get in a good position for your hips and lower back. Here are some suggestions for helping you sit better, if you have to sit:

- Take regular breaks. Get up and walk around. If you drive for work, pull over to walk and stretch.

- Make sure that in your seat (at work or at the dinner table) your hips and knees have a minimum of a 90-degree bend. Ideally your hips will be higher than your knees so that the joints are open more than 90 degrees. Sit on the corner of the chair, not the edge.

- Try variety. A sit-stand desk would be a good choice, but if it's not an option, cross one leg over, then cross the other, sit in a four position (one ankle crossed over the other knee), sit with legs crossed yoga style, squat if your attire and office allows it.

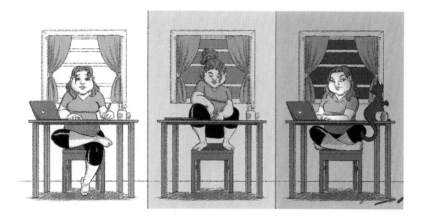

- When sitting at home, try to incorporate more variety. Sit in different positions on the floor, which will be working all sorts of muscles to get you up and down off the floor as an added bonus. Getting up and down off the floor is good for our health and a skill we don't want to lose. Consider sitting on the floor to eat dinner, play with kids, or to put your shoes on.

Are Your Tight Hamstrings Causing Your Back Pain?

Now you know that when we refer to tight hamstrings, it does not necessarily mean that you need to stretch them all day because they are tight and strong. Very often, they can be tight and weak. Do you get a sensation of cramping when you do hamstring exercises? That's a sign the muscle is weak. On a positive note, it's a sign that you are getting the muscle to fire, but the muscle doesn't feel strong enough to do the work so it cramps.

Those tight muscles running down the back of your leg are likely pulling on your pelvis all the time, keeping it tucked under and lengthening the muscles of the low back. Then we go to move to pick something up off the floor. We could squat to reach it or hinge at the hip on one leg while floating the other leg up behind to counterbalance. Those would be good options.

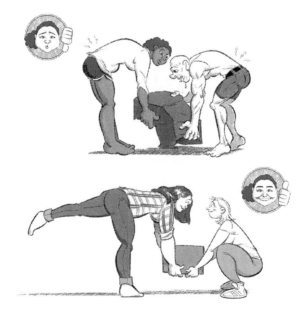

More often than not, however, we tend to round forward in the spine while our butt tucks under. This reveals the tight hamstrings in action, putting pressure on the low back. Our hamstrings are so tight they are limiting our mobility and range of motion at the hip joint. Our hips can't move, so our back does the work. Then, over time, our back starts to ache. We have to both strengthen and lengthen those pesky hamstrings for the health of our spine. It's a moral imperative.

To help alter patterns of picking items up, try the Tipping Bird described earlier in our eccentric contraction Movement Break. Also, consider wagging your tail. Huh? Did you know that you can move your tailbone like you can move all your vertebrae? At least you should be able to, but in order to feel it, you may have to do a little digging. The best place to move your tailbone is in the shower. Remember in *Dirty Dancing* when Johnny takes Baby to the water to practice the lift because it was the best place? It's kind of like that only less romantic. Next time you take a shower, find your tailbone with your finger. You don't actually have to go too deep into any crevices to find it, but you will be descending into crack territory.

Once you find it, engage your pelvic floor (think Kegel). You should be able to feel the tailbone wiggle a little bit. Think of the range of motion you can get from the first joint of your pointer finger. It's not a big movement, but you should feel something. You'll need to engage and release to experience movement. The pelvic floor muscles will have to engage toward the back. When we think Kegel, we often limit ourselves to part of the muscle toward the front. Once you can feel the little guy moving, you don't always need to actually find your tailbone to recreate this exercise. It's worth finding the first time to ensure you get the movement right. If that's a little too intimate for you right now, that is okay.

The tailbone is really the last bone of our spine. If something in the body is meant to have mobility, we want to keep it mobile. Since everything is connected, if our pelvic floor is too tight or too slack, that disturbs the positioning of the tailbone, which is connected to the sacrum, which is connected to the lumbar spine. One influences the other. If you've ever broken your tailbone or had coccyx pain, you know firsthand how much your tailbone matters. Simply sitting becomes miserable. Tight hamstrings that tuck the tailbone under all day often result in lack of tone in the pelvic floor, and the combination could contribute to your back pain.

Now, Spread 'Em!

Ninety-eight percent of the hip replacements in the United States are successful, but if and when they fail, they are more likely to fail in women.[63] This shows more research is required to help us understand what women need when it comes to hip replacements. Doctors think this failure is due in part to women having smaller bones and therefore needing smaller implants, so the ball that is replaced in the socket is smaller. Biomechanical engineer and blogger Katy Bowman thinks the cause might be mechanical, which could explain needing the hip replaced in the first place. It might be as simple as women standing with their feet too close together.[64] In general, women have wider pelvises than men but stand with their feet together rather than hip distance apart, which equates to more pressure and torque where the femur (thigh bone) and pelvis meet.

So, women, what have you got to lose? Spread those legs a little.

---

63 Ryan Jaslow, "Hip Replacements More Likely To Fail in Women, Says Study," *CBS News*, February 18, 2013.

64 Katy Bowman, "Girly Hips," *Katy Says…* (blog), February 19, 2013, https://www.nutritiousmovement.com/girly-hips/.

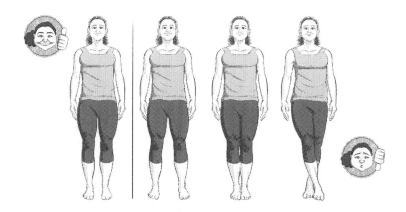

Don't take them as wide as shoulder width, but check in when you stand to see how wide or un-wide your legs are. Your feet should not touch or be wider than your entire pelvis. Hip distance apart does not mean as wide as your pelvis. For ideal alignment, your feet, knees, and legs should line up with where your femur comes into your pelvis. Where do your feet land? It's not that any of these positions are specifically harmful or ways we should not stand. They are all okay, however, it is patterns that cause trouble in our body. So if you have a tendency to kick a hip out or stand with crossed legs, it is worth noticing and adjusting some of the time.

Your Knees

What are the knees doing in the Happy Hips & Low Back section? Most knee pain develops over time from natural wear and tear, poor posture, or faulty alignment. Osteoarthritis has long been nicknamed "the wear and tear" arthritis. Though knees are often susceptible to acute injuries like a sporting injury or falling in a groundhog hole, which definitely require a doctor's attention, chronic knee issues more often than not developed from what was originally an issue in the hip or ankle. If you have knee issues, many of the exercises for Happy Hips and Happy Feet may help.

While our knee joint has some rotation between the lower leg and the knee, for the most part it really is primarily a hinge joint, bending the leg back and straightening. The joints on either end (hip and ankle) are considerably more complicated. They flex and extend like the knee, but they also rotate, and the ankle pronates and supinates. Both those end joints operate in more planes of motion than the knee. If either the ankle or the hip is a little bit out of its neutral home position, that alteration will constantly place a sense of tug or torque on the knee joint. Fallen arches or flat feet can make the knees buckle in like we are knock-kneed. A rotation at the hip that turns the leg inward (think pigeon-toed) forces the knee to point inward too. The poor knee is often forced to play along with the larger hip or the super-mobile ankle.

Additional Tips to Support the Spine

There are many ways you can create a better position for your spine throughout the day. Here are a few suggestions.

Rise up. Put a triangle wedge in your car seat to prop your hips higher. You achieve a better angle in the hip joint when the hips are higher than the knees, and it will help tip your pelvis forward so that you sit more on your sitz bones, not rolled off behind them. You could add this to any chair you sit in. You could also use a higher desk chair or stand-sit desk. Your hips should be higher than knees any time you sit, or else your pelvis and back won't have a chance. At a minimum, you want 90 degrees at your hips and knees when sitting, but in an ideal world that angle is larger. Get those hips up. If nothing has worked to reduce chronic back pain and you sit for long intervals during the day, you must reduce the amount you sit or at least increase the angle.

Stay in motion. The less we move, the more pain worsens. Find stretches that feel good on your back. Move more in general. Regular movement can reduce back pain. It may have to be subtle at first or at times, but that is okay. Subtle, small steps are the secret to reducing pain. You'll probably progress the most with understated movements. Take short walks. Squat more. If you watch TV, get up and squat during commercials. Think about what you are feeling and where you are feeling it, and start with small progressions to bigger movements as your body becomes ready. A small study of Japanese workers found that those with back pain who rested had more issues with chronic back pain than those who remained active.[65] Immobility is rarely beneficial to the body, and limited movement is better than none. This might include gentle passive mobilization provided by a physical therapist or gentle exercises. When in pain or inflamed, move what you can. More often than not, pain will increase over time without movement.

Find alignment. Alignment is not a perfect answer because our body is not supposed to be stuck in a definitive stature. We should be able to move in all sorts of ways, and we shouldn't have to be in neutral all the time to be happy. Life doesn't always happen in neutral. However, finding better alignment can be a tool to decrease low back pain. If you think about your posture every hour for one minute, that's more than before. Try to increase over time. Put reminders in your phone to consider how you hold yourself in space. When sitting, try to lengthen out of your slump. When standing, play with all sorts of weight shifts in the body. Can you push your hips back or forward, untuck your tailbone, move your ribs forward and back? Play with the alignment of the body to try to find your middle, where your head is over your ribs, ribs are over your hips, and hips are over your heels. Can you find a center point where you don't feel the need to slouch, no part of your body feels tense, and you feel well balanced? "No" or "I'm not sure" is always fine. Do you kick one

---

65 Carrie DeVries, "Bed Rest Is Not the Best for Beating Back Pain," *Spine-health*, *Veritas Health*, June 28, 2016, https://www.spine-health.com/blog/bed-rest-not-always-best-bet-beating-back-pain.

hip out to the side throughout the day? How does shifting your weight side to side alter what you are feeling? Do you get more pain or less pain in certain positions? Start taking stock of your body in space throughout the day.

The floor is your friend. Get down on the floor. This isn't just good for your spine, it's also good for your whole body. More importantly, it's a "move it or lose it" kind of thing. If you are currently unable to get up and down off the floor, try to build up to that as a goal. If you still have the capability, get on the floor every day to put your socks and shoes on in order to maintain that ability. Get down to play with kids in your family. Maybe even have dinner there.

Variety is key. Find different ways to sit, walk, move, and exercise. Variety is important to healing the body. Remember when your mom would respond to your nasty faces by saying that if you made the face for too long it might get stuck like that? With the body, it's true. Embrace one shape too often, and your muscles will adjust so that position becomes easier to maintain. It's thoughtful of them, but everything else gets harder. Our muscles can be a little shortsighted.

Hydrate regularly. If you have chronic back pain or regularly pull your back, hydrate. This is especially important before a flight, a long car ride, or any period where you might have to sit for an extended timeframe. The thick, lumbar fascia does well when hydrated. Fuel it constantly.

Be gentle and relax. When you lie down in bed tonight, check in with your body. Are you actually relaxed? Can you relax something more: quads, shoulders, forehead, jaw, glutes? Consider the Constructive Rest position (see Movement Break on page 195) and take a few deep breaths there. Be gentle with yourself. Trust what you feel. Listen to your body. If you are in pain, your body has been trying to get your attention. Try not to judge what you do or don't feel. Move with caution at first. Very often when we are in pain, we are hesitant to do certain moves. Treat yourself to a massage. A good massage therapist can reduce back pain.

Lift from your legs, not your back. When you squat to lift something, if you come up with the weight in your toes, the burden is still on your back. As you come up, keep the weight over your heels. Imagine pushing the floor away with your heels (you were just practicing this in the squats). Just because you are doing a squatting motion doesn't mean your back isn't doing the work. The squat should come from strength in your legs. When in doubt, stick it out. As you squat, try not to let your tailbone tuck under by the tug of those pesky, tight hamstrings. Do this anytime you lift something, even if it's small and light.

In addition to these small adjustments and daily habits, you can also support your spine by integrating the following exercises into your fitness routine.

Exercises for the Back

See **Calf Stretch** on page 187

Double Calf Stretch.

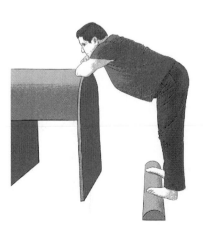

Standing, place balls of feet on half foam roller or rolled-up yoga mat. Hinge forward at hips and place hands on a table or supportive ledge with arms extended. Line up hips directly above heels. Tip tailbone up toward ceiling and hold stretch for four to five breaths.

Make sure feet are parallel on the foam roller and the "knee pits" are pointing backwards. You do not have to bend forward too far. Ease in. You are looking for a stretch in the back of your body (calves and hamstrings ideally). The pelvis and back should be neutral, not rounded.

Pelvic Tilts.

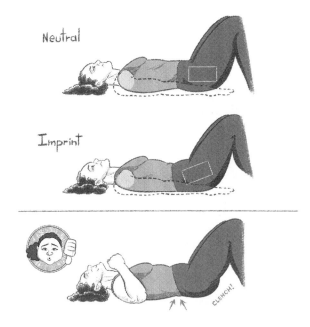

Lie on back with knees bent.

Start with a neutral pelvis with a slight arch in low back. Inhale to hold.

Exhale: Rock to imprint, pressing the low back gently against the floor.

Watch out for: 1) Squeezing the butt. You should move from your abs like a pair of suspenders that connects your ribs and hips is shortening. 2) Being too aggressive. Move slowly and feel that all the work comes from your abs. Try not to jam your back into the floor. 3) Moving too much. Less is more here. Try to make sure only the pelvis and low back are moving, not the ribs, neck, or head.

Cat Stretch.

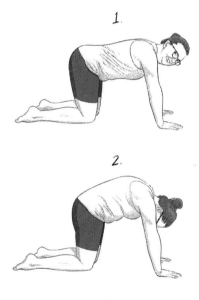

Return to start ☺

Start on all fours with knees hip distance apart and hands shoulder width apart. Keep your abs gently engaged or reconnect with them on every exhale.

Inhale: Stick your tailbone out and slide your shoulders down. Look up, extending the spine.

Exhale: Tuck the tailbone between your legs (like you've been a bad dog), round the back like a Halloween cat, and let your head hang.

Inhale: Stay and try to stretch deeper with the breath.

Exhale: Unwind to extend the spine and return to start position.

Repeat three to ten times.

Spinal Rotation.

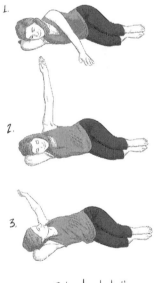

Return to start ☺

Lie on your side with hips stacked. Knees and hips each have a 90 degree angle. Use a pillow under your head. Both arms reach out in front.

Inhale: Stay.

Exhale: Bring your top arm up to the ceiling and continue rotating back toward the floor, looking toward your moving hand. Feel a stretch through the front of your chest.

Inhale: Stay.

Exhale: Return.

NOTE: Try not to let your hips and legs rock back when you open the chest.

Sciatica Tip:

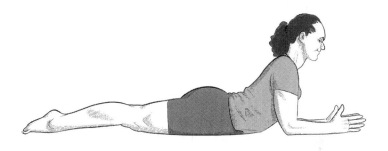

Try this position for sciatica relief. Lie down on your stomach on a firm surface with legs straight behind you on the floor, prop yourself up on your forearms, and hold for a few deep breaths. A sciatic relief position should make you feel relief almost immediately. It should not increase pain at all. If you get into a position that seems to aggravate the sciatica, get out of it. In my experience, this position works for the majority of people (but not everyone). If this position is right for your body, you will feel the pain in your legs diminish.

Exercises for the Hips

Monster Walk.

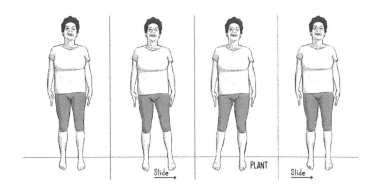

Can be done with or without an exercise flex band. If using a band, place or tie it around ankles ensuring nothing is dangling down to trip on. Feet are parallel and about hip width apart. Keeping tension on the band and weight in heels, start at one end of the mat (hips square to the front), move sideways one step at a time by sliding one foot out, planting it, and then bringing the other foot in, always keeping tension in the band. Take five to ten steps sideways, then five to ten steps back the other way. Repeat three to four times in each direction.

Advanced Monster Walk.

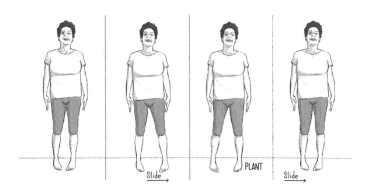

After doing the monster walk with legs and feet parallel, try a second set, keeping the legs rotated in. Rotate at the thighs so the knees angle in, making sure the movement is at the hip and not created from torquing the knee or twisting the foot. If it bothers the knee, skip this.

Hip Flexor Stretch.

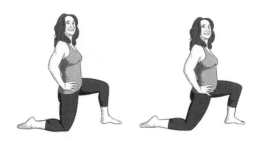

Kneel (if that is an option), bring one foot forward like you are proposing, then inch the front foot forward a little so that it is not directly under your knee. Stay tall through the trunk, tuck your tailbone (imprinting), and lean forward from the front knee, bringing the knee over the foot. You should feel the stretch in the front of your back leg. Zip the jeans and engage your back glute to feel more. Hold for 15 to 30 seconds and repeat on the other side. Breathe throughout.

Four Stretch.

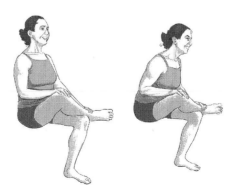

(Not an option for those with hip replacements.) Sitting in a chair, cross one leg over the other so that one ankle is resting above the other knee. If this is enough of a stretch, stay here. If you want more, hinge (do not round) forward at the hips.

Clam Shell.

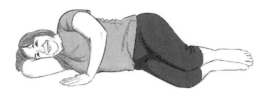

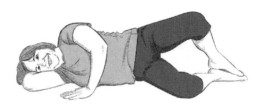

Lie down on one side with legs bent and hips wider than 90 degrees. Feet and knees start together. Lift the top knee while keeping the feet together. Try not to rock the hip back. Lower the leg. Repeat up to 12 times on each side and try to imagine you are moving through molasses.

CHAPTER 10: HAPPY NECK & SHOULDERS

Following the trampoline incident that resulted in whiplash, I could not move my neck without pain for weeks. This is the trap many of us fall into, pushing our bodies during a workout or physical task when we are exhausted. Eventually, the body will cry uncle and throw in the towel as mine did on my last flip. A friend of mine (actually the same friend who hurt both his Achilles tendons when he switched to minimalist shoes for running) turned 50 and mentioned that the thing he missed most about being a kid is how he was able to bounce back effortlessly after a fall. Over the winter, he had gone sledding with his college-aged son and slipped on the ice; his legs came up from under him and he fell spread eagle on his back. He didn't bound back up to race down the hillside. He said he felt the shock reverberate through every bone in his entire body, and he had to stop and assess whether or not he could even get back up.

That's exactly how it was for me as I lay as still as I could on that trampoline. Fortunately, my neck healed (mostly). Once we have an injury, it can require ongoing or possibly occasional maintenance. Ever since my failed flip, now and again my neck gets cranky and requires attention. When it is aggravated, my range of motion becomes limited. It feels like I slept on it wrong. Tiny movements reduce the pain, so I search for whatever movement, no matter how subtle, I can find in that moment. I turn my head a quarter inch to the right and do little, tiny head nods like I'm saying "yes" or "no." Slowly, that small move progresses to a larger, more encouraging nod. Movement spreads throughout the body.

An Unstable Joint

We live in a world of stress, tense shoulders, and stiff necks. According to the Bureau of Labor Statistics, while back problems are more prevalent, people miss more work due to shoulder injuries. The shoulder is a complex, unstable joint, which is part of the reason so many of us experience pain in our neck and shoulders. Frozen shoulder, whiplash, rotator cuff injuries, and bursitis are the most common shoulder ailments. Understanding how the joint works can help you realize which daily activities may be creating or exacerbating pain. For example, are your shoulders tense and shrugged up to your ears right now? Relax them.

The shoulder joint is described as a ball and socket joint. While that is technically true, it looks more like a golf ball sitting on a tee. There's not much socket. Since the bones are not deeply set into each other, the joint provides more mobility but less stability than any other joint in the body. With great mobility comes increased responsibility to stabilize. Mobile joints come with added vulnerability. Instead of the bones providing stability, we must rely on a complex combination of muscles, tendons, and ligaments working together dynamically creating stability during motion. In the shoulder, the musculature helps create the joint.

Our scapula, or shoulder blade, has 16 muscles tugging it in various directions. Visualize a triangle with multiple rubber bands coming off of the three sides. If you pull one rubber band tight, the triangle moves in that direction and the other rubber bands get longer or shorter to accommodate the movement. If one band is pulling forcibly all the time, it will affect the other bands, either creating tautness in certain muscles or causing a weakness in muscles that are too small to resist the pull.

The shoulder may be best known for its ball and socket joint, but it is actually made of three separate joints that work together with the ribcage, thoracic spine (mid-back), and neck in order to allow the arm to move. The joints involved are the *glenohumeral joint* (where the head of the arm bone and side of the scapula meet), *acromioclavicular joint* (where the top of the scapula and the breastbone meet), and *sternoclavicular joint* (where your breastbone and sternum meet). All of them are mouthfuls, I know. On Facebook, the shoulder's relationship status would definitely be "it's complicated."

The scapula should lie reasonably flat against the ribcage, gliding along it to reposition itself during spinal, arm, and shoulder movements. It basically floats on the ribs, suspended with muscles. When all those muscles work properly, this is a great arrangement because the scapula must glide, slide, and move in order for us to have a full range of arm movements. If the muscles restrict the scapula, we lose motion in our arm. With proper tracking of the scapula during movement, the arm should be able to lift to 180 degrees. Envision making a snow angel. Our arms should have the freedom to move from hanging at our sides by our legs, out to our sides like a cross, and up directly overhead along our ears. (I'll wait while you check your range of motion.)

Proper tracking is called *scapulohumeral rhythm*. It's not a modern dance move, but you can think of it like a dance. The scapula and arm move like partners, one leading the other. If the scapula doesn't follow or stumbles, then the arm bone bumps into the top of the shoulder blade (the *acromion*) when we try and raise it up. This cramping of space creates compression on all the other muscles, tendons, and ligaments squished and rubbing against each. Everything in there is still trying to move, but it's as if instead of four lanes of traffic merging into three to get through a smaller tunnel, the four lanes forced their way through as if four lanes still existed. All the cars made it through the other side, but scratched, dented, and much worse for wear. Repetitive friction leads to future rotator cuff injuries.

Movement Break: Shoulder Series

Movement One: Good Alignment

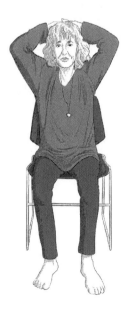 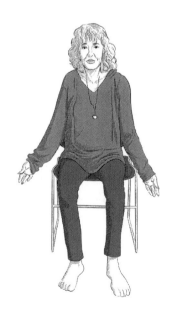

- Sit in a good posture and place your hands on top of your head. Elbows should land a little forward of head. Try not to force them wider.

- Shrug and drop your shoulders a few times to get tension out of your muscles.

- Then try to keep shoulders relaxed and lower one arm at a time.

This movement is intended to improve the placement of the scapula at rest. This is the optimal alignment of your shoulders and scapula.

Movement Two: Spider Fingers

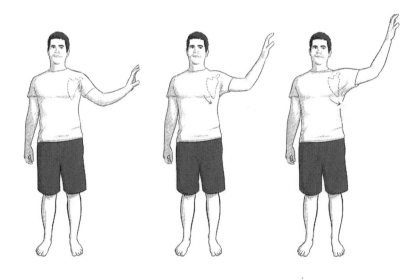

Stand next to a wall with your hand on the wall about the height of your chin and slightly forward of your body. You are not facing the wall; the wall is next to the side of whichever arm you are working.

- Walk your fingers up the wall. As you do this, try to prevent your shoulder from shrugging and instead feel the scapula rotate up to follow the arm movement.

- Walk the hand back down the wall.

- Repeat four to five times on each arm.

- Do a second set facing the wall, crawling both arms up at the same time.

In this movement, the wall helps take the weight of the arm off the shoulder so that the scapula and arm can dance together more freely.

Movement Three: Scapulohumeral Rhythm

- Standing or sitting, start with your arms hanging at your side.

- Inhale to lift your arms up like you are making a snow angel as high as you can without forcing it.

- Exhale to lower the arms on the same path.

- NOTE: Can your arms go all the way up and down without your shoulders shrugging up? Is your range of motion limited? Can you feel if your scapula is moving with you? If it is, you'll have a full range of motion.

Posture and alignment play a major role in the happiness of our shoulders. In a world of sitting and spending our days slumped forward over technology, we tend to have really tight pec muscles (the muscles in the front of your chest). More often than not, these muscles are super tight and pull the arm bone forward and out of alignment. Exacerbating this, some people have a push-up obsession, which only works the pecs more. This is a good place to think about eccentric contractions to make muscles long and strong. Whether you do push-ups on the wall or on the floor (on your knees or toes), consider slowing down the descent of the push-up but pressing up at a normal speed. You'll challenge the eccentric movement of the muscle so that it can stay long and strong, emphasizing the movement that promotes elongating the muscle. That way, you will keep it strong but less tight, and you'll be doing your entire shoulder girdle a service.

The Shoulder-Rib Connection

When we have shoulder pain, like any pain, we need to consider the body as a whole. Maybe the cause of the pain didn't originate in the shoulder. Maybe something is going on somewhere else in the body. This holds true for most pain, but the shoulder joint, like the knee, is especially prone to having its root cause stem from another part of the body.

Which brings us to the shoulder-rib connection. The ribcage isn't part of the shoulder joint, but the placement of the ribs in space and in alignment with the rest of the body is related to shoulder health and stability. The shoulder blade needs to be able to settle against the ribs and move freely and smoothly. If the scapula doesn't rest against the ribs or has a bumpy ride as it moves, the shoulder joint may be affected. If you have poor posture and often slump forward (kyphosis), you can do exercises for your shoulder all day long, but if you do them without correcting where the ribs and thoracic (middle back) are in space, you can be creating more strain or compression on the muscles and tendons that stabilize the joint.

Similarly, a tight psoas (the muscle running from your thigh to multiple vertebrae in the low back) can tug your spine, and therefore your ribs, forward into a rib thrust, which can result in limited movement between the spine and the shoulders. The pain may be in the shoulder, but the original culprit may exist elsewhere in the body. The reason we have to look at the body globally when we have an injury is that only focusing on the injured location is limiting in the midst of pain. It's possible that area requires some rest. Attention elsewhere could help resolve the problem area. If you have pain in your neck and shoulders, make sure you have read the section on posture.

I came to fully comprehend how connected our ribs, shoulder, and everything in our body are when I had costochondritis. Years ago I caught a cough like no other. My boyfriend, Matt, was the original carrier of this wretched croup. It involved six weeks of a hacking, full-body, wake-you-up-in-the-middle-of-the-night beast that shook my chest and scratched my throat. Triggered by an unpleasant virus going around, after six weeks of hacking in addition to larynx spasms, I developed agonizing rib pain. Had the pain not been completely linked with movement, I would have presumed I was having a heart attack. Shooting pains radiated down my arm. Rolling out of bed produced tortured moans. The pain was so severe it could only be a cracked rib, I presumed. X-rays showed nothing, which meant I had costochondritis: inflammation of the cartilage between the ribs, often caused from a prolonged or hard cough.

The doctor suggested I take Aleve. I capitulated and was forced to modify some of my exercises because basic movements hurt too much. A month later the world was looking good again. Nearly pain-free, I sneezed. This time, the pain took my breath away and nothing audible filtered its way passed my lips. Breathless, I wrapped my good arm around my ribs as if giving myself a hug, attempting to self-soothe and hold myself together. A pint of ice cream was consumed for medicinal purposes.

This round was even worse. For about two days, driving hurt, breathing was torture, opening the refrigerator felt like someone was stabbing me (which tragically meant gaining access to ice cream was difficult). Movement felt like the enemy; I was terrified of sneezing and couldn't get comfortable in bed. I went back to the doctor, sure that I had done something worse. They must have missed the crack in my ribs. Clearly, some bone was detached and dangling inside me. Nope. It was still *just* costochondritis. Nothing was cracked or dislocated, yet my pain was prohibitive. Doctors don't get up in arms about costochondritis, but movement is how I earn a living. Movement is also what keeps me sane. They doubled my dose of Aleve (something I don't recommend because of the stomach side effects), suggested using a muscle relaxing ointment and ice, and stated that I should not do ANYTHING that aggravated it. That was laughable. Everything aggravated it. The once simple act of inhaling and exhaling made me wince. I was told no Pilates, running, or swimming for at least three weeks or until all symptoms were completely gone.

This was a disaster. Movement is my drug of choice. "This isn't permanent. This could be worse," I told myself while reaching for a bar of dark chocolate with my one good arm. With whiplash, I had figured out my limitations quickly. Now, I was gripped with fear, constantly bracing for the next sneeze, cough, or deep breath that would send me back to the doctor claiming my lung had collapsed only to be told I had a papercut. Generally, I've learned to appreciate pain in my body because I always learn something from it. This time, I was a living example of how everything in the body is connected, and when one part of the body moves, it affects another. The connection between my ribs and my fingertips had never been apparent to me. Since ribs and the muscles and cartilage between them are linked with every single action we take, no matter how tiny, opening a door or turning a steering wheel hurt. Pain forced me to become obnoxiously self-aware.

Within days of taking the double dose of Aleve, I felt like it had torn a hole in my stomach. After over a week of icing my ribs and trying to remain still, I was leaps and bounds better but remained anxious that something simple would set me back to square one. Fear of pain limited my movement for over a year. At first, there were moves I wouldn't do. Arm exercises like push-ups or pull-ups were out the question. Nerves could have held me hostage in my own body. Instead, I pushed myself cautiously.

For an entire year, I explored movements I could manage. Working with Pilates, a massage therapist, and a chiropractor equipped me to expand my capabilities. When the body is in pain, careful and cautious experimentation with different types of therapies and movement is essential. If one modality doesn't work, others still might, or a combination may be best. Every therapeutic avenue I attempted helped me improve, even if it was to learn not to do something at that moment. Everything was a piece of the puzzle that I could not replicate perfectly for someone else's body. It took over a year to feel like the pain from costochondritis was truly gone, but I still take heed of any sensation I get around my ribs when I'm exercising. I'll rein movement in when I get a signal that seems foreboding. Having returned to all former exercises, except pull-ups, my understanding and communication with my body has improved.

One cough didn't give me costochondritis. One move did not make it go away. Everything I did was a piece of a year-long puzzle to help me feel normal. As often is the case in life, it is about finding balance when in pain. Push too hard or too soon, and you may have a setback. Do nothing, and you'll definitely experience a setback. Through experimentation and listening to subtle signals, you can start to learn what your body requires. As frustrating as it may be, it takes time. Change comes incrementally. That is why movement can be less appealing than a pill, but it is far more effective.

While I never want to have costochondritis again, I now know that if my ribs are ever riddled with pain in the future, I will be able to overcome it. We never know the end result, but there is no reason to believe the outcome will be a lifetime of pain. If I continued to allow my fear of pain dictate my movements, in a few years, in addition to having costochondritis, I'd probably have chronic neck and shoulder pain. Left unchecked, pain spreads. My tendency to keep my pain a secret was not helpful. People all over the world are living in fear from their experience with costochondritis. Many find it debilitating for a time. You are never in pain alone. Every human experiences pain.

Tips for Resolving Costo

Experimentation is key. I can't swear by one method. While immobilization is counterintuitive to me and goes against most of what I say in this book, I did reduce my movement to allow my soft tissue to heal. Attempting to immobilize the ribs and arm while in pain helped, but this is not a permanent solution. While I was in pain, I moved whatever I could, whether that was my neck or my feet. You can always move something, and that provides hope. Any movement is better than none because any movement benefits the irritated bit since it's all connected. Besides, as long as we are still breathing, we cannot fully immobilize the ribcage. I kept moving but ceased any and all movement that hurt, including all upper body arm exercises, for three weeks. Here are other tactics that I found helpful:

- Massage

- Muscle rub ointments each night

- Regular icing

- Aleve (helpful for inflammation but not for the stomach)

- Pilates

- Walking

- Bracing the ribs before a cough, sneeze, or laugh

- A good chiropractor

- Exploring breath patterns that feel okay

Once you can move again, it is important to maintain mobility in the mid-back and throughout the ribs. Deep breathing can help with this, but we can also try to move the ribcage by sliding it side to side like a typewriter or trying to make circles with the ribs.

Common Shoulder Pain Culprits

Shoulder pain often develops over time with wear and tear. You may note a specific moment in time when pain became unbearable suddenly, but chances are the injury was building beneath the surface.

Rotator Cuff (RC) Tear

Unless you are an athlete or a baseball pitcher, this is probably not an acute injury. Even if you did something that suddenly tore the rotator cuff muscles or tendons, chances are that posture or a repetitive motion has worn them down over time. The rotator cuff refers to one or multiple of four muscles in your shoulder. While you don't need to know the name of all the muscles, you can remember them with SITS (subscapularis, infraspinatus, teres minor, supraspinatus). One of the causes of repetitive strain on the RC muscles or tendons is that, with our shoulders rolled forward or squeezed back, we limit the space for these muscles and tendons, causing constant abrasion by our bones. Over time, this wears on them. You might have done an exercise or movement for years without a problem and now it's bothering you. You don't blame that repetitive motion because you've always done it, but it is likely that any repetitive motion has been wearing away at the RC muscles and tendons if the joint isn't in good alignment (see the posture section again on page 130). These muscles are small but do a lot of hard work. They don't require hard, muscle grinding exercise. What they require (but often do not get) is space within the joint in order to move and glide freely.

Frozen Shoulder (AKA Adhesive Capsulitis)

I like the scientific name here, because it sounds right. Something is stuck. Frozen shoulder is the perfect example of a chronic injury because it builds over time, often stemming from a prior injury or surgery when we limited our arm movement. While you may not notice until your movement is very limited, frozen shoulder doesn't happen overnight. It usually involves immobility and pain in the shoulder joint, and it can improve and go away with time. Move what you can. Everything is connected. Moving one part supports and influences another.

Tendinitis

This can happen to multiple tendons within the shoulder joint; a rotator cuff tendon or biceps tendon are most common. Overuse and a wearing down of the tendon are usually the most common causes. (Are you noticing the pattern to how the shoulder develops pain?) Tendinitis is inflammation. Sometimes people are diagnosed with tendinitis when they really have tendinosis (degeneration of the tendon) or tendinopathy (a disease or disorder of the tendon). If anti-inflammatories are not helping, tendinopathy might be the cause.

All of these common habits are relievable, and even reversible, especially if you catch them early. Most of them originate with poor posture and learned movements that put pressure on an area that shouldn't have pressure. The good news about a learned behavior like posture is that it can be changed. Phew!

The Neck and Its Woes

The neck has similar problems to the shoulders and low back. It provides mobility but has minimal stability. Many of the muscles operating our neck are teeny-tiny in comparison to the rest of our body. The longest human neck, according to the *Guinness Book of World Records*, is 15.75 inches. This length did not come naturally. It was created by fitting copper coils around a woman's neck, a tradition of the Padaung and Kareni tribes in Myanmar. Luckily, this trend has been losing popularity, as an elongated neck eventually can't hold the head and can become fatal if the coils are removed. It serves as a good example of when we should ask if our fashion statements are worth the strain on our bodies.

Our necks are rather delicate. They have smaller muscles and bones and very little protection. Plus, they have to hold our 11-pound heads all day long. Some of the most common neck injuries include:

Whiplash

This is typically an acute injury, most often associated with car accidents. People eye roll when someone complains about whiplash, but it really does hurt and can be debilitating for a while. Whiplash is when our head gets thrown forward or backward quickly, causing tears or pulls in the muscles or tendons. It's literally a strain in our neck.

Repetitive Strain

Even something as simple as sleep can cause neck strain. We've all woken up and felt like we've slept on our neck wrong and spent the rest of the day with a stiff neck. Often neck strain, like a lot of chronic pain, originates with faulty posture. We tend to be a society of forward-jutting heads and necks. Looking down at books, phones, or our feet lengthens the muscles of the back of our neck, keeping them in a constant state of strain and tension. When your neck aches, it's usually the back of the neck. Other parts of your neck may hurt, but more often than not the poor, overworked back-of-the-neck is experiencing tension. See the Turkey Trot exercise on page 235 and the section on posture on page 130 to try to reduce neck strain.

Degenerative Disc Disease (DDD)

Over time, we all have wear and tear on our discs throughout our back, but some people never experience pain. The neck and low back are the most likely to have DDD, but it can happen anywhere in the spine. DDD isn't a disease; it's the term for damaged discs. The discs between all our vertebrae act as shock absorbers all day long from the moment we lift our head off the pillow. They allow for fluid, flexible movement throughout the spine. Damage is caused suddenly by an injury or over time through chronic use. As our discs get damaged from life, they can repair and build up scar tissue, but that scar tissue is never quite as strong as the original disc. It's unclear why some people experience pain and others do not as our discs age. Here's some good news: as bad as this one sounds—like a disease that is going to get worse over time—there are plenty of people whose pain doesn't get worse. A diagnosis of degenerative disc disease is not a life sentence for chronic pain.

Forward Heads

As a society, we tend to jut our heads forward. While technology and books exacerbate the problem, the fact that we have eyes on the front of our head is part of the problem too. We lead with our heads. We are oriented forward.

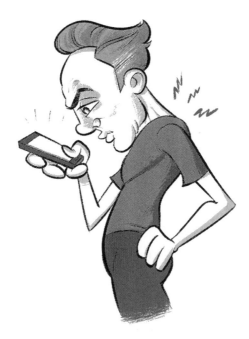

If your head juts forward and your shoulders roll forward, you are likely to experience discomfort in your upper back and neck.

Every movement that follows begins with strain and tension where some muscles and tendons are overstretched and others are overtight. It's this kind of "faulty" movement that ultimately leads to common neck and shoulder injuries.

Think for a second. Do you feel or have you felt like you have a knot right in between your neck and shoulders? The muscles you are feeling are usually your upper trapezius or your rhomboids, which get sad, tired, and overstretched when you round forward. Still, they are desperate to do their job of holding your head and shoulders back throughout the day. They are losing the constant tug-of-war and basically knot themselves in desperation. While no one really knows what that knot in the muscles is caused by, it is believed to be an over-contraction of the muscle due to overuse and faulty biomechanics. Some believe they are myofascial trigger points. Others believe they are irritated nerves and that nothing is wrong with the muscles. No matter the cause, the way to resolve them is likely the same. Strengthen and stretch appropriately to seek balance between the muscles and consider your alignment throughout the day.

Movement Break: Turkey Trot

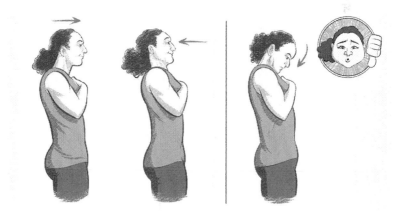

You look funny doing this one, but if it alleviates pain, the turkey trot neck exercise is worth the strange looks. The pulling back motion of this exercise can give muscles of our neck and upper back a bit of relief and place them in a more comfortable position momentarily. Plus, this is a simple, subtle exercise. And if you've ever had bad neck pain—whiplash or even simply woken up with a stiff neck—you know small moves may be all you can handle.

- Sit or stand tall with your best posture. NOTE: If you do this exercise in a slump without sitting tall, it will not be beneficial and could exacerbate pain. If you cannot sit or stand with proper posture yet, skip this one for now.

- Look straight ahead. Try not to let your chin drop.

- Pull your head backwards like you are trying to give yourself a double chin. Focus on moving the head back without tucking the chin to the chest.

- Move the head forward. Rein in how far forward you can go.

- Try the same concept with the head against an object, standing against a wall, or lying on the floor. If you are against the floor or the wall, gently apply pressure as if you are pushing your head into sand. You don't need to cram it.

- For more guidance, place one hand on your belly and one on your chest. Check in that your posture is good, maybe even slightly pushing your breastbone toward your chest hand.

- As you move your head, make sure the rest of the spine doesn't move. Your belly and chest beneath your hands should remain stacked on top of each other and still.

Feel relief when you pull back? If not, maybe this one isn't for you right now.

Hopefully, the turkey trot can give you some relief during the day, but what about relief at night? We spend about eight hours in bed each night. That's a lot of time that we are supposed to be healing and recuperating. If you need relief at night too, you might need to re-evaluate your pillow choices.

When the Pillow is the Bad Guy

It is possible your pillow is adding to your neck or shoulder pain. There is no one-size-fits-all when it comes to pillows. It is possible to prefer being too propped up, which pushes your head and neck forward at night the way it was stuck all day. There is very little research on whether pillows are beneficial or not, so experimenting with different pillows, configurations of the pillow, or positions may help resolve your issues. Consider rolling a towel under your neck at night while back sleeping. If it feels good, use it as a tool. If not, don't worry. Also, consider experimenting with your head and shoulders (not just your head) on the pillow. See how that feels.

If you've been having chronic neck and shoulder issues, try making a change in your sleeping arrangements. You have nothing to lose. Sometimes what we presume is good for us isn't, or what once worked for us no longer does. If you asked me what kind of pillow would be the best, I'd have guessed a feather pillow, but in one of the few studies done on pillows (that arguably had some flaws), feathers fared the worst and latex pillows the best.

Before jumping into the exercises, keep in mind that many neck and shoulder muscles are small, and micro-movements are beneficial. Big sweeping gestures will often bypass the tiny muscles. When your neck or shoulders are injured, take a step back to explore where can you get some movement, no matter how trite it may seem. Can you find a small range of motion that feels doable or ideally good? Start there and move forward.

Neck & Shoulder Exercises

Hanging Arm Circle.

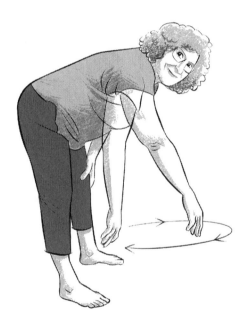

Hinge forward at the waist and bend knees into a shallow squat. Rest one hand on thigh for support and let the other arm hang down. Allow the hanging arm to circle freely in the shoulder joint. Do several circles, and then switch directions. Repeat on the other arm. Try to keep the back as flat as possible while circling the arm.

Ear to Shoulder/Upper Trapezius Stretch.

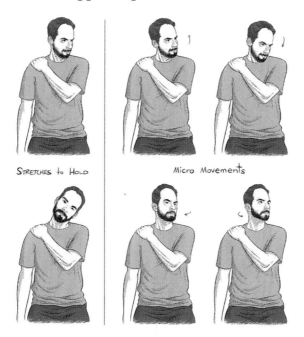

STRETCHES to HOLD   Micro Movements

From a seated or standing position, tip your head to the right, dropping your ear toward your shoulder. Place your right hand on your left shoulder, and gently draw the shoulder down to create more stretch. Hold for four to five breaths, then repeat on the other side.

Chin toward Underarm/Levator Scapula Stretch. From a seated or standing position, turn your head about 45 degrees to the right, then drop your chin toward your collarbone (it will look like you are trying to sniff your armpit). You can add a little more stretch by placing your right hand behind head and drawing the chin down more. Hold for four to five breaths, then repeat on other side.

Yes/No. Turn head about 45 degrees to the right. Lengthen posture (as if a string was drawing head toward ceiling). Then begin making small, controlled "yes" motions for 15 seconds followed by "no" motions with your head for 15 seconds. Repeat toward the other side.

Pilates Arm Circles.

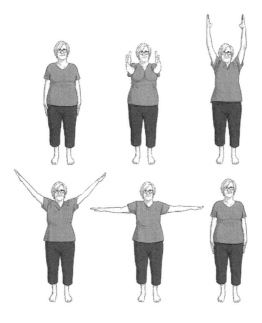

Sitting tall, on the inhale, lift arms in front of you and straight overhead. On the exhale, sweep the arms out to the sides like you are making a snow angel. Repeat four to five times, then reverse directions.

Snow Angels.

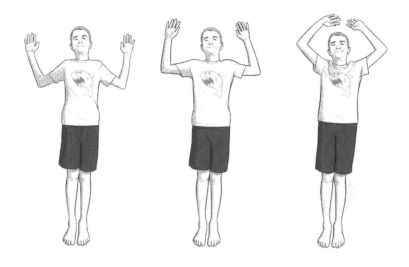

Lie on your back with knees bent and feet flat on the floor. Begin with arms on a mat, with elbows out to the sides, and hands rotated palms up like you are making the shape of a goalpost with your arms. To start with, try to keep all these points flat at the same time (shoulder blades, elbows, wrists, hands, fingers, ribs). At first, it will be challenging to keep them all down. That can be the exercise for a while. Never be forceful. You do not have to add movement. After you've mastered keeping everything flat at the same time, try to keep even pressure against the floor with all those points and trace snow angels while the elbows remain bent. When you have mastered these skills on the ground, try them standing against a wall.

Zeppelin.

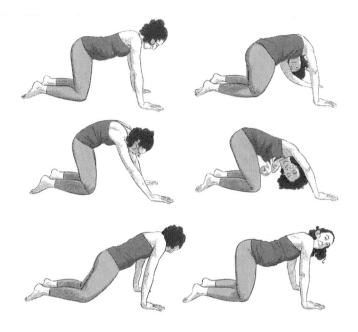

This is a great movement exploration exercise that will improve strength at your shoulder (and hip!) joints while also improving core and upper back strength. Begin with knees under hips and hands under shoulders. Without moving hands and knees, move the rest of your body and explore how many different positions you can get in, what kinds of weight shifts you can make, and what patterns you can create with your spine. When you get more comfortable, you can experiment with bringing one arm off the floor and exploring movement on three points instead of four.

Final Foundations for Fighting Pain

Your pain is real. Every signal your brain sends you is your reality. When stuck in a pain loop, we have to take control of the wheel and work to rewire the brain so that it learns new tricks. We need to remind ourselves that we can move with less discomfort and that we have options.

Ask for personal attention from your doctor, physical therapist, or any practitioner you are working with one-on-one. While there are standards that can help people heal and get out of pain, in the end, everyone is different and needs to be treated as such. Keep seeking answers. Someone may express an idea in this book in a different way and that is when you will have your "ah-ha" moment. Someone may have an entirely new idea for you or a way that helps you understand your body even better. This isn't the end of your discovery and return to movement. This is just the beginning.

As you go off into the world with the intent of moving more, trust yourself. You know your body better than anyone. Movement does not and should not have to hurt. It is okay for you to tell anyone instructing you that something hurts and that you'd rather not work through excessive pain. We all experience pain differently, and whatever you feel is okay and beneficial feedback for you and your practitioner. Be clear about what you feel and what you are not comfortable doing. Trust that you may intuitively know what is happening in your body. You never have to feel bad about saying a particular movement hurts or sitting out an exercise in a group class. When something doesn't feel right in your body, ask for an explanation as to why the pain sensation is helping the process or ask for a different movement. Because the entire body is interconnected, the ability to move any one part is helpful to the whole.

Traditional exercise isn't the only option. Learning to alter daily patterns can make huge changes and help us get out of painful positions. Movements that properly strengthen your core and postural muscles not only aid in the mind-body connection but also promote overall health. Be willing to explore micro-movements, weight shifts, changes throughout daily tasks, and breathing patterns. Pain will never disappear from your life forever. You will have moments of physical pain that creep up, return, or find you anew throughout life. Pain is meant to help you and serves as an important guide.

When I visit my grandma, she is always willing to let me video her doing a movement to fill the feeds of my social media. The videos I post of her are some of my most popular, partly because she is adorable and endearing but also because she is impressive. We all want to be 92 and still moving. Our lives are made better by movement. We can retain independence when we move.

Like wrinkles, pain is a part of our story. We can relate to others with and through our pain. Eventually, we can even laugh about pain or how we ended up in pain. It helps keep us alive. How we respond to that pain makes the difference. Movement is the best response. You were born to move. Explore movement with an open mind. Listen to what you feel, and remember that no movement is too small. If you have been living with pain, you are a fighter. Keep fighting, and know that whatever you can do today is enough.

RESOURCES

Free Resources

» Subscribe to the Keep Moving Blog at www.personaleuphoria.com/keep-moving for more tips and stories.

» You can find a number of short workouts and explanations of exercises on my YouTube channel: EuphoriaPilates at www.youtube.com/user/EuphoriaPilates/

» Some specific videos that may help you are:
Positions to Reduce Neck Pain on Ab Exercises
Posture Play: Try Not to Pop the Chest

Paid Resources

If you are interested in purchasing any of the Workshops for Wellness series, please visit: www.PEEPsinMotion.com. Use code KEEPMOVINGREADER to get $10 off the Happy Feet, Happy Hips & Low Back, and Happy Neck & Shoulders online workshops. Each workshop has the exercises in this book, plus additional exercises and tips. If you found this book helpful, there is even more guidance to be found in the online programs!

ACKNOWLEDGEMENTS

You. The reader. I'm endlessly appreciative that you picked my words to spend time with. According to author John Cheever, writing without a reader is like a kiss—you can't do it alone. It thrills me that you picked *Keep Moving* off the shelf or placed it in your online cart. Matt Atwater, who let me ramble about movement on long walks and always supports my dreams. Plus, he is the best dealer of oxytocin. My mom, Deb Bax, who reminds me not everyone is actually interested in fascia, and if I want to make people care, I have to make it interesting and then is willing to read multiple versions of a chapter about fascia. My dad, Bill Downie, and stepfather, Anthony Bax, because they love me, which gives me strength. Cate Vallone, my mentor, friend, and PEEPs in Motion co-creator—without her, the Happy Body Series would not exist, and there would be a lot less fun in the world. She is my movement buddy. Plus, she never thinks fascia is boring. My clients who trust me with their most precious commodity—their bodies. They show up, do the work, and let me learn from them every day. Their curiosity, engagement, and trust make me a better teacher. The readers who suffered on this first draft and told me to keep going: Julie Wernau and my mom (who has read this more than anyone). My sister, Helen Odell, who took a ton of work off my plate to enable me to focus on this project. My brother, Will Downie, whose edits made me laugh out loud and showed me what I didn't know I didn't know. Nicole Ferrari Mitchell, the first friend I trusted with these stories, whose ideas helped improve them and who encouraged me to continue. Ethan Harper, who I hoped would one day illustrate something I wrote since the day I met him in junior high. His mind is filled with extraordinary characters. Jeanette Downie who was always available to bounce around ideas and deserves credit for "Take Steps." Molly Forrester who took a major task off my hands. Pat Kennedy, Gail Dimaggio, and David Frye—the most extraordinary teachers who kept me spellbound and encouraged. The Paper Raven peeps. Morgan Gist MacDonald and the entire team were guides through uncharted water, helping me fulfill a dream, a passion, and an adventure. Joy Xiang, Karen Furr, Jesus Cordero, Darcy Gist, Claudia Sanchez, Amanda Kuebler, Victoria Klein, Rachela Brisindi, Shena Sabens, and Joe Walters provided guidance and reassurance along the way. My great-grandma, Lavina Leonide Bradshaw Downie; my grandmas; my stepmother, Ellen Downie; and my mom give me confidence, courage, and character. Everyone I reached out to with a question about pain seemed eager to talk and supportive of this project. There are a number of experts out there who care and are motivated to help. I hope you find the right one for you.

WORKS CITED

Ahmad, Asma Hayati, and Rahimah Zakaria. "Pain in Times of Stress." *The Malaysian Journal of Medical Sciences* 22 (Dec 2015): 52–61. https://www.ncbi.nlm.nih.gov/pmc/articles/PMC4795524/.

Alami, Sophie et al. "Management of Pain Induced by Exercise and Mobilization during Physical Therapy Programs: Views of Patients and Care Providers." *BMC Musculoskeletal Disorders* 12 (2011): 172. https://doi.org/10.1186/1471-2474-12-172.

Amabile, Amy H., John H. Bolte, and Saskia D. Richter. "Atrophy of Gluteus Maximus Among Women with a History of Chronic Low Back Pain." *PLOS ONE* 12, no. 7 (2017). https://doi.org/10.1371/journal.pone.0177008.

The American Academy of Pain Medicine. "AAPM Facts and Figures on Pain." Accessed March 2018. https://www.painmed.org/patientcenter/facts_on_pain.aspx.

American Physical Therapy Association. "APTA History." January 10, 2017. http://www.apta.org/History/.

American Physical Therapy Association. "Many PT Programs Describe Their Pain Management Education as Not 'Adequate.'" PT in Motion, March 3, 2015. www.apta.org/PTinMotion/News/2015/3/3/PTPainEducation/.

American Society of Addiction Medicine. "Opioid Addiction 2016 Facts & Figures." Accessed July 2018. https://www.asam.org/docs/default-source/advocacy/opioid-addiction-disease-facts-figures.pdf.

Anderson, Barton E., and K. C. H. Bliven. "The Use of Breathing Exercises in Treatment of Chronic, Nonspecific Low Back Pain." *Journal of Sport Rehabilitation* 26 no. 5 (2017): 452–58. https://doi.org/10.1123/jsr.2015-0199.

Anita. "Not Just Skin Deep: Neurons Detect Pleasurable Touch." *Knowing Neurons*, February 18, 2013. https://www.knowingneurons.com/2013/02/18/not-just-skin-deep-neurons-detect-pleasurable-touch/.

Banth, Sudha, and Maryam Didehdar Ardebil. "Effectiveness of Mindfulness Meditation on Pain and Quality of Life of Patients with Chronic Low Back Pain." *International Journal of Yoga* 8, no. 2 (Jul–Dec 2015): 128–33. https://www.ncbi.nlm.nih.gov/pmc/articles/PMC4479890/.

Baron, Kelly Glazer, Kathryn J. Reid, and Phyllis C. Zee. "Exercise to Improve Sleep in Insomnia: Exploration of the Bidirectional Effects." *Journal of Clinical Sleep Medicine* 9, no. 8 (2013): 819–24. http://dx.doi.org/10.5664/jcsm.2930.

BBC News. "'Green' Exercise Quickly 'Boosts Mental Health.'" Updated May 1, 2010. news.bbc.co.uk/2/hi/health/8654350.stm.

Bell, Vaughan. "The Unsexy Truth About Dopamine." *The Guardian*, February 2, 2013. www.theguardian.com/science/2013/feb/03/dopamine-the-unsexy-truth.

Bhandari, Smitha, ed. "Sensory Processing Disorder." *WebMD*. Updated January 8, 2017. https://www.webmd.com/children/sensory-processing-disorder#2.

Bi, Xia et al. "Pelvic Floor Muscle Exercise for Chronic Low Back Pain." *Journal of International Medical Research* 41, no. 1 (2013): 146–52, https://doi.org/10.1177/0300060513475383.

Biello, David. "Inside the Debate About Power Posing: A Q&A with Amy Cuddy." Ideas.Ted.com, February 22, 2017. https://ideas.ted.com/inside-the-debate-about-power-posing-a-q-a-with-amy-cuddy/.

Bogduk, Nikolai, and Gunnar Andersson. "Is Spinal Surgery Effective for Back Pain?" *F1000 Medicine Reports* 1, no. 60 (2009). http://doi.org/10.3410/M1-60.

Bowman, Katy. "Alignment Is Not Posture." *Katy Says...* (blog), May 21, 2014. https://www.nutritiousmovement.com/alignment-is-not-posture/.

———. "Girly Hips." *Katy Says...* (blog), February 19, 2013. https://www.nutritiousmovement.com/girly-hips/.

Boyle, Kyndall L., Josh Olinick, and Cynthia Lewis. "The Value of Blowing Up a Balloon." *North American Journal of Sports Physical Therapy* 5, no. 3 (Sept 2010): 179–88. https://www.ncbi.nlm.nih.gov/pmc/articles/PMC2971640/.

Boyle, Michael. "Is 'Rotation Training' Hurting Your Performance? a.k.a. 'Is Rotation Even a Good Idea.'" *Sports Rehab Expert*, 2007. https://www.sportsrehabexpert.com/public/97.cfm.

Breus, Michael J. "Better Sleep Found by Exercising on a Regular Basis." *Psychology Today*, September 6, 2013. https://www.psychologytoday.com/us/blog/sleep-newzzz/201309/better-sleep-found-exercising-regular-basis-0.

Brooks, Michael. "Researchers Have a Gut Feeling—Could Chronic Pain Be Caused by Bacteria?" *New Statesman*, March 19, 2015. https://www.newstatesman.com/lifestyle/2015/03/researchers-have-gut-feeling-could-chronic-pain-be-caused-bacteria.

Buettner, Dan. "How To Live To Be 100+." Filmed September 2009 in Minnesota. TED video, 19:33. www.ted.com/talks/dan_buettner_how_to_live_to_be_100.

Carroll, Aaron E. "To Lose Weight, Eating Less Is Far More Important Than Exercising More." *The New York Times*, June 15, 2015. www.nytimes.com/2015/06/16/upshot/to-lose-weight-eating-less-is-far-more-important-than-exercising-more.html.

Catlin, Brian, and John Lyons. "Etymology of Abdominal Visceral Terms." Edited by Rand Swenson. Dartmouth Medical School, 2008. www.dartmouth.edu/~humananatomy/resources/etymology/Shoulder_arm.htm.

Centers for Disease Control and Prevention. "Sleep and Sleep Disorders." Updated February 22, 2018. https://www.cdc.gov/sleep/index.html.

Chan, Brenda L. et al. "Mirror Therapy for Phantom Limb Pain." *The New England Journal of Medicine*, 357 (2007): 2206–07, http://doi.org/10.1056/NEJMc071927.

Chen, Yi-Wen et al. "The Effect of Tai Chi on Four Chronic Conditions—Cancer, Osteoarthritis, Heart Failure and Chronic Obstructive Pulmonary Disease: A Systematic Review and Meta-Analyses." *British Journal of Sports Medicine* 50, no. 7 (2016): 397–407. https://bjsm.bmj.com/content/50/7/397.info.

The Children's Hospital of Philadelphia. "Amplified Musculoskeletal Pain Syndrome (AMPS)." 2014. https://www.chop.edu/conditions-diseases/amplified-musculoskeletal-pain-syndrome-amps.

Christian, Lisa M. et al. "Stress and Wound Healing." *Neuroimmunomodulation* 13, no. 5–6 (2006): 337–46. http://doi.org/10.1159/000104862.

Connor, Steve A. "The People Who Can't Feel Pain: Scientists Discover Cause of Rare Inherited Condition That Turns Off Brain Sensors." *Independent*, May 25, 2015. www.independent.co.uk/life-style/health-and-families/health-news/the-people-who-cant-feel-pain-scientists-discover-cause-of-rare-inherited-condition-that-turns-off-10274604.html.

Cook, A. C. et al. "Early Mobilization Following Carpal Tunnel Release. A Prospective Randomized Study." *Journal of Hand Surgery* 20, no. 2 (1995): 228–30. https://doi.org/10.1016/S0266-7681(05)80057-9.

Costa, Allison B. "The Dangers of the 'No Pain, No Gain' Mentality in Modern Exercise." Digital Commons at University of Rhode Island, May 2015. https://digitalcommons.uri.edu/srhonorsprog/413/.

Craig, A. D. 2002. "How Do You Feel? Interoception: The Sense of the Physiological Condition of the Body." *Nature Reviews Neuroscience* 3: 655–66. https://doi.org/10.1038/nrn894.

———. "Interoception: The Sense of the Physiological Condition of the Body." *Current Opinion in Neurobiology* 13, no. 4 (Aug 2003): 500-05, https://doi.org/10.1016/S0959-4388(03)00090-4.

Crettaz, Benjamin et al. "Stress-Induced Allodynia—Evidence of Increased Pain Sensitivity in Healthy Humans and Patients with Chronic Pain after Experimentally Induced Psychosocial Stress." *PLOS ONE* 8, no. 8 (2013). https://doi.org/10.1371/journal.pone.0069460.

Daily Mail. "Duke University Scientists Find Women Need More Sleep than Men." *News.com.au,* December 21, 2013. www.news.com.au/lifestyle/health/duke-university-scientists-find-women-need-more-sleep-than-men/news-story/145ac5019468614c170432eba0a78977.

Daily Mail Reporter. "Gentle Jogging Once a Week 'Can Add Six Years to Your Life.'" Updated May 4, 2012. http://www.dailymail.co.uk/health/article-2138869/Jogging-increases-life-expectancy-Gentle-jogging-week-add-6-years-life.html.

DeVries, Carrie. "Bed Rest Is Not the Best for Beating Back Pain." *Spine-health. Veritas Health*, June 28, 2016. https://www.spine-health.com/blog/bed-rest-not-always-best-bet-beating-back-pain.

Doheny, Kathleen. "Here's How Much Running Is Healthiest for You, According to One Study." *Health*, February 2, 2015. https://www.health.com/fitness/when-it-comes-to-jogging-easy-does-it-study-suggests.

Doyle, Kathryn. "Switch to Minimalist Running Shoes Tied to Injuries, Pain." *Reuters*, January 9, 2014. https://www.reuters.com/article/us-running-shoes-injury/switch-to-minimalist-running-shoes-tied-to-injuries-pain-idUSBREA081CS20140109.

Duke University School of Medicine. "Duke-Led Study Finds that Moderate-to-Vigorous Workouts Reduce Mortality." Duke University Health System, March 22, 2018. https://medicine.duke.edu/medicinenews/duke-led-study-finds-moderate-vigorous-workouts-reduce-mortality.

Dusenbery, Maya. "'Everybody Was Telling Me There Was Nothing Wrong.'" *BBC*, May 29, 2018. https://www.bbc.com/future/story/20180523-how-gender-bias-affects-your-healthcare.

Dvoskin, Rachel. "Sweeter than Cocaine." *Scientific American*, April 1, 2008. https://www.scientificamerican.com/article/sweeter-than-cocaine/.

Eligon, John, and Serge F. Kovaleski. "Prince Died from Accidental Overdose of Opioid Painkiller." *The New York Times*, June 2, 2016. www.nytimes.com/2016/06/03/arts/music/prince-death-overdose-fentanyl.html?_r=0.

Elkins, Lucy. "Who Really Needs More Sleep—Men or Women? One of Britain's Leading Sleep Experts Says He Has the Answer." *Daily Mail*, January 26, 2010. www.dailymail.co.uk/health/article-1246029/Who-REALLY-needs-sleep--men-women-One-Britains-leading-sleep-experts-says-answer.html.

English, Bella. "Health Walk Inspired by President Adams." *Boston Globe*, April 20, 2014. https://www.bostonglobe.com/metro/regionals/south/2014/04/19/john-adams-health-walk-quincy-continues-early-president-advocacy-exercise/ZcZ8xmn3kc8ZMRBPPKO75H/story.html.

Ergotron. "New Survey: To Sit or Stand? Almost 70% of Full Time American Workers Hate Sitting, but They Do It All Day Every Day." Prnewswire.com, July 17, 2013. www.prnewswire.com/news-releases/new-survey-to-sit-or-stand-almost-70-of-full-time-american-workers-hate-sitting-but-they-do-it-all-day-every-day-215804771.html.

European Medical Alliance. "Unconscious Proprioception." Updated June 10, 2018. www.europeanmedical.info/blood-pressure/unconscious-proprioception.html.

Evans, Subhadra et al. "Yoga for Youth in Pain: The UCLA Pediatric Pain Program Model." *Holistic Nursing Practice* 26, no. 5 (Sep–Oct 2012): 262–71. http://doi.org/10.1097/HNP.0b013e318263f2ed.

Fenwick, Steven A., Brian L. Hazleman, and Graham P. Riley. "The Vasculature and Its Role in the Damaged and Healing Tendon." *Arthritis Research* 4, no. 4 (Feb 2002): 252–60. https://doi.org/10.1186/ar416.

Fernández-de-las Peñas, César et al. "Manual Physical Therapy Versus Surgery for Carpal Tunnel Syndrome: A Randomized Parallel-Group Trial." *The Journal of Pain* 16, no. 11 (Nov 2015): 1087-94, https://doi.org/10.1016/j.jpain.2015.07.012.

Folk, Jim, and Marilyn Folk. "Psychological Stress Can Make Pain Worse." *Anxietycentre.com.* Updated July 21, 2018. https://www.anxietycentre.com/anxiety/research/psychological-stress-can-make-pain-worse.shtml.

França, Fábio Renovato et al. "Segmental Stabilization and Muscular Strengthening in Chronic Low Back Pain: A Comparative Study." *Clinics* 65, no. 10 (2010): 1013–17. https://doi.org/10.1590/S1807-59322010001000015.

Freedman, Michael D. et al. "The Role of the Lumbar Multifidus in Chronic Low Back Pain: A Review." *PM&R* 2, no. 2 (Feb 2010): 142–46. https://doi.org/10.1016/j.pmrj.2009.11.006.

Friedrichsdorf, Stefan J. et al. "Chronic Pain in Children and Adolescents: Diagnosis and Treatment of Primary Pain Disorders in Head, Abdomen, Muscles and Joints." Edited by Carl L. von Baeyer. *Children* 3, no. 4 (2016): 42. https://doi.org/10.1016/j.jpain.2012.03.009.

Gaskin, Darrell J., and Patrick Richard. "The Economic Costs of Pain in the United States." *The Journal of Pain* 13, no. 8 (Aug 2012): 715–24. https://doi.org/10.1016/j.jpain.2012.03.009

Globerson, Eitan, and Israel Nelken. "The Neuro-Pianist." *Frontiers in Systems Neuroscience* 7 (Jul 2013). https://doi.org/10.3389/fnsys.2013.00035.

Gmuca, Sabrina et al. "Presenting Manifestations of Amplified Musculoskeletal Pain Syndrome in Males versus Females." *American College of Rheumatology Abstracts* 69 (2017). https://acrabstracts.org/abstract/presenting-manifestations-of-amplified-musculoskeletal-pain-syndrome-in-males-versus-females/.

Goeij, Moniek et al. "Systematic Inflammation Decreases Pain Threshold in Humans in Vivo." *PLOS ONE* 8 no. 12 (2013). https://doi.org/10.1371/journal.pone.0084159.

Gordon, Susan J., Karen A. Grimmer-Somers, and Patricia H. Trott. "Pillow Use: The Behavior of Cervical Stiffness, Headache and Scapular/Arm Pain." *Journal of Pain Research* 3 (2010): 137–45. https://www.ncbi.nlm.nih.gov/pmc/articles/PMC3004642/.

Gouin, Jean-Philippe et al. "Marital Behavior, Oxytocin, Vasopressin, and Wound Healing." *Psychoneuroendocrinology* 35, no. 7 (2010): 1082–90. https://doi.org/10.1016/j.psyneuen.2010.01.009.

Gregoire, Carolyn. "How Our Sense of Touch Affects Everything We Do." *Huffington Post*, January 20, 2015. https://www.huffingtonpost.com/2015/01/20/neuroscience-touch_n_6489050.html.

Hamblin, James. "Why One Neuroscientist Started Blasting His Core." *The Atlantic*, August 24, 2016. www.theatlantic.com/science/archive/2016/08/cortical-adrenal-orchestra/496679/.

Hanson, Patrick et al. "Anatomical Differences in the Psoas Muscles in Young Black and White Men." *Journal of Anatomy* 194, no. 2 (Feb 1999): 303–07. https://doi.org/10.1046/j.1469-7580.1999.19420303.x.

Hardison, Mark E., and Shawn C. Roll. "Mindfulness Interventions in Physical Rehabilitation: A Scoping Review." *The American Journal of Occupational Therapy* 70, no. 3 (May–Jun 2016). https://doi.org/10.5014/ajot.2016.018069.

Harvard University. "A History of fMRI." Massachusetts General Hospital. Athinoula A. Martinos Center for Biomedical Imaging. Accessed January 2018. www.nmr.mgh.harvard.edu/history-fMRI.

Healey, Kellie C. et al. "The Effects of Myofascial Release with Foam Rolling on Performance." *Journal of Strength and Conditioning Research* 28, no. 1, (Jan 2014): 61–68, https://doi.org/10.1519/JSC.0b013e3182956569.

Hegarty, Stephanie. "The Myth of the Eight-Hour Sleep." *BBC News*, February 22, 2012. https://www.bbc.com/news/magazine-16964783.

———. "What Phantom Limbs and Mirrors Teach Us About the Brain." *BBC News*, December 5, 2011. https://www.bbc.com/news/magazine-15938103.

Herbert, Beate M., and Olga Pollatos. "The Body in the Mind: On the Relationship Between Interoception and Embodiment." *Topics in Cognitive Science* 4, no. 4 (Oct 2012): 692–704. https://doi.org/10.1111/j.1756-8765.2012.01189.x.

Herbert, Beate M. et al. "Interoception across Modalities: On the Relationship between Cardiac Awareness and the Sensitivity for Gastric Functions." *PLOS ONE* 7, no. 5 (2012). https://doi.org/10.1371/journal.pone.0036646.

Higgs, Robert. "When You Gotta Go, You Should: Holding It and Holding It Can Lead to Health Consequences." *Cleveland.com*. Advance Local Media. Updated April 21, 2009. https://www.cleveland.com/healthfit/index.ssf/2009/04/go_when_you_gotta_holding_it_a.html.

Holpuch, Amanda. "Black Patients Half as Likely To Receive Pain Medication as White Patients, Study Finds." *The Guardian*, August 10, 2016. www.theguardian.com/science/2016/aug/10/black-patients-bias-prescriptions-pain-management-medicine-opioids.

Hu, Hai et al. "Is the Psoas a Hip Flexor in the Active Straight Leg Raise?" *European Spine Journal* 20, no. 5 (May 2011): 759–65. https://doi.org/10.1007/s00586-010-1508-5.

Inacio, Maria C. S. et al. "Sex and Risk of Hip Implant Failure: Assessing Total Hip Arthroplasty Outcomes in the United States." *JAMA Internal Medicine* 173, no. 6 (2013): 435–41. https://doi.org/10.1001/jamainternmed.2013.3271.

Jarrett, Christian. "Mirror Neurons: The Most Hyped Concept in Neuroscience?" *Psychology Today*, December 10, 2012. https://www.psychologytoday.com/us/blog/brain-myths/201212/mirror-neurons-the-most-hyped-concept-in-neuroscience.

Jaslow, Ryan. "Hip Replacements More Likely To Fail in Women, Says Study." *CBS News*, February 18, 2013. www.cbsnews.com/news/hip-replacements-more-likely-to-fail-in-women-says-study/.

Kankaanpää, Markku et al. "Back and Hip Extensor Fatigability in Chronic Low Back Pain Patients and Controls." *Archives of Physical Medicine and Rehabilitation* 79, no. 4 (Apr 1998): 412–17. https://doi.org/10.1016/S0003-9993(98)90142-3.

Kannus, Pekka. "Immobilization or Early Mobilization After an Acute Soft-Tissue Injury?" *The Physician and Sportsmedicine* 28, no. 3 (Jun 2015): 55–63. https://doi.org/10.3810/psm.2000.03.775.

Kaufman, Elizabeth L., Jenna Tress, and David D. Sherry. "Trends in Medicalization of Children with Amplified Musculoskeletal Pain Syndrome." *Pain Medicine* 18, no. 5 (May 2017): 825–31. https://doi.org/10.1093/pm/pnw188.

Keck Medicine of USC. "Thoracic Surgery." 2018. https://surgery.keckmedicine.org/treatments-services/usc-thoracic-surgery/.

Khan, Serajul I., and John A. Burne. "Reflex Inhibition of Normal Cramp Following Electrical Stimulation of the Muscle Tendon." *Journal of Neurophysiology* 98, no. 3 (Sep 2007): 1102-07. https://doi.org/10.1152/jn.00371.2007.

Kimball, Molly. "Can a Shot of Pickle Juice Alleviate Muscle Cramps?" *Nola.com.* Advance Local Media, March 30, 2015. https://www.nola.com/healthy-eating/2015/03/pickle_juice_for_muscle_cramps.html.

Kissass Facts Fact Encyclopedia. "25 Interesting Facts About Human Hormones." November 15, 2014. www.kickassfacts.com/25-interesting-facts-about-human-hormones/.

Koerth-Baker, Maggie. "First Shoes Worn 40,000 Years Ago." *Live Science.* Purch, June 5, 2008. https://www.livescience.com/4964-shoes-worn-40-000-years.html.

Krueger, James M., David M. Rector, and Lynn Churchill. "Sleep and Cytokines." *Sleep Medicine Clinics* 2, no. 2 (2007): 161–69. https://www.ncbi.nlm.nih.gov/pmc/articles/PMC2605347/.

Layne, Jennifer E., and Miriam E. Nelson. "The Effects of Progressive Resistance Training on Bone Density: A Review." *Medicine & Science in Sports and Exercise* 31, no. 1 (Jan 1999): 25–30. https://doi.org/10.1097/00005768-199901000-00006.

Lee, I-Min et al. "Effect of Physical Inactivity on Major Non-Communicable Diseases Worldwide: An Analysis of Burden of Disease and Life Expectancy." *The Lancet* 380, no. 9838 (July 2012): 219–29. https://doi.org/10.1016/S0140-6736(12)61031-9.

Lenoir, Magalie et al. "Intense Sweetness Surpasses Cocaine Reward." Edited by Bernhard Baune. *PLOS ONE* 2, no. 8 (2007). https://doi.org/10.1371/journal.pone.0000698.

Lewis, Jordan Gaines. "Smells Ring Bells: How Smell Triggers Memories and Emotions." *Psychology Today*, January 12, 2015. www.psychologytoday.com/us/blog/brain-babble/201501/smells-ring-bells-how-smell-triggers-memories-and-emotions.

Library of Congress. "What Is the Strongest Muscle in the Human Body?" Everyday Mysteries, July 31, 2017. www.loc.gov/rr/scitech/mysteries/muscles.html.

Liebenson, Craig. "Vleeming's Active SLR Test as a Screen for Lumbopelvic Dysfunction." *Dynamic Chiropractic* 21, no. 5 (Feb 2003). https://www.dynamicchiropractic.com/mpacms/dc/article.php?id=9052.

Litzy, Karen. "201: Busting Tendinopathy Myths with Dr. Jill Cook" *Healthy, Wealthy, Smart Podcast.* February 29, 2016.

Louw, Adriaan, et al. "The Clinical Application of Teaching People About Pain." *Physiotherapy Theory and Practice* 32, no. 5 (2016): 385–95. https://doi.org/10.1080/09593985.2016.1194652.

Louw, Adriaan, et al. "The Efficacy of Pain Neuroscience Education on Musculoskeletal Pain: A Systematic Review of the Literature." *Physiotherapy Theory and Practice* 32, no. 5 (2016): 332–35. https://doi.org/10.1080/09593985.2016.1194646.

Ma, C. Benjamin. "Pain and Your Emotions." Edited by David Zieve and Brenda Conaway. MedlinePlus. U.S. National Library of Medicine, September 7, 2017. https://medlineplus.gov/ency/patientinstructions/000417.htm.

Mandal, Ananya. "Dopamine Functions." News-Medical.net. Updated August 23, 2018. https://www.news-medical.net/health/Dopamine-Functions.aspx.

McColm, Jan. "A Hug a Day." *Endeavors*. UNC-Chapel Hill, January 1, 2004. http://endeavors.unc.edu/win2004/hugs.html.

The Medical Dictionary. s.v. "lateral raphe." The Free Dictionary. Farlex and Partners, 2009. https://medical-dictionary.thefreedictionary.com/lateral+raphe.

Mikkelson, David. "Muscles to Smile and Frown." Snopes, February 1, 2008. https://www.snopes.com/fact-check/happiness-is-only-grin-deep/.

Miller, Becky. "Sleep & Muscle Recovery." Livestrong, August 14, 2017. https://www.livestrong.com/article/155363-sleep-muscle-recovery/.

Mullington, Janet M. et al. "Sleep Loss and Inflammation." *Best Practice & Research, Clinical Endocrinology & Metabolism* 24, no. 5 (2010): 775–84. https://doi.org/10.1016/j.beem.2010.08.014.

Nash, C. E. et al. "Injured Limbs Recover Better with Early Mobilization and Functional Bracing Than with Cast Immoblization." *The Journal of Bone & Joint Surgery* 87, no. 5 (2005): 1167.

National Institutes of Health. "Brain Basics: Understanding Sleep." Office of Communications and Public Liaison. Updated July 6, 2018. https://www.ninds.nih.gov/ Disorders/Patient-Caregiver-Education/Understanding-Sleep.

National Institutes of Health. "Charcot-Marie-Tooth Disease Fact Sheet." National Institute of Neurological Disorders and Stroke, July 6, 2018. https://www.ninds.nih.gov/ Disorders/Patient-Caregiver-Education/Fact-Sheets/Charcot-Marie-Tooth-Disease-Fact-Sheet.

National Sleep Foundation. "Do Women Need More Sleep than Men?" Accessed March 2018. https://www. sleepfoundation.org/sleep-news/do-women-need-more-sleep-men.

NBC News. "Experimental Treatment Regrows Muscle in Injured Men's Legs." April 30, 2014. www.nbcnews.com/ health/health-news/experimental-treatment-regrows-muscle-injured-mens-legs-n94101.

New Scientist. "Body Illusions: Rubber Hand Illusion." March 18, 2009. https://www.newscientist.com/article/ dn16809-body-illusions-rubber-hand-illusion/.

Newcomb, Tim. "German Diver Sets Breath-Holding Record: 22 Minutes, 22 Seconds." *Time Magazine Newsfeed*, June 5, 2012. newsfeed.time.com/2012/06/05/german-diver-sets-breath-holding-record-22-minutes-22-seconds/.

Nu Image Medical. "HGH: A Possible Cure for Sleep Disorders?" 2014. https://nuimagemedical.com/hgh/hgh-a-possible-cure-for-sleep-disorders.

O'Keefe, James H., and Carl J. Lavie. "Run for Your Life…at a Comfortable Speed and Not Too Far." Independent Organizations at the University of Virginia, January 11, 2013. indorgs.virginia.edu/MuscleClub/OKeefe_JH_article1%2B2. pdf.

Olson, Eric J. "Lack of Sleep: Can It Make You Sick?" Mayo Clinic. MFMER, June 9, 2015. www.mayoclinic.org/diseases-conditions/insomnia/expert-answers/lack-of-sleep/faq-20057757.

Parker-Pope, Tara. "Women's Heart Symptoms Often Blamed on Stress." *The New York Times blog*, October 13, 2008. https://well.blogs.nytimes.com/2008/10/13/just-stress-more-often-diagnosed-in-women/.

Pavlova, M. et al. "Disentangling the Sleep-Pain Relationship in Pediatric Chronic Pain: The Mediating Role of Internalizing Mental Health Symptoms." *Pain Research and Management* 2017. https://doi.org/10.1155/2017/1586921.

Peak Performance Physical Therapy. "Factors That Affect Your Balance and Risk of Falling." Accessed November 2017. www.peakptfit.com/factors-that-affect-your-balance.

Physiopedia. "Low Back Pain and Pelvic Floor Disorders." January 10, 2018. https://www.physio-pedia.com/index.php?title=Low_Back_Pain_and_Pelvic_Floor_Disorders&oldid=182218.

Physiopedia. "Pain Neuroscience Education (PNE)." March 9, 2016. https://www.physio-pedia. com/index.php?title=Pain_Neuroscience_Education_ (PNE)&oldid=135525.

Pickering, Mark, and James F. X. Jones. "The Diaphragm: Two Physiological Muscles in One." *Journal of Anatomy* 201, no. 4 (Oct 2002): 305–12. https://doi. org/10.1046/j.1469-7580.2002.00095.x.

Pomeroy, Ross. "To Be Fit and Healthy, Live Like Benjamin Franklin." *Real Clear Science*, September 23, 2012. https://www.realclearscience.com/blog/2012/09/the-ben-franklin-diet.html.

Provine, Robert. "The Science of Laughter." *Psychology Today*. Sussex Publishers. Updated June 9, 2016. https://www. psychologytoday.com/us/articles/200011/the-science-laughter.

Ramin, Cathryn Jakobson. *Crooked: Outwitting the Back Pain Industry and Getting on the Road to Recovery*. New York: Harper, 2017.

Rantala, Jussi, and Jukka Rasaimo. "Proprioception" University of Tampere, Finland. Accessed November 2017. www.uta.fi/sis/tkt/hui/schedule/HUI2011-3-proprioception. pdf.

Rettner, Rachael. "How Your Brain Works on Autopilot." Live Science, June 9, 2010. https://www.livescience. com/6557-brain-works-autopilot.html.

Reynolds, Gretchen. "Moderation as the Sweet Spot for Exercise." *The New York Times blog*, June 6, 2012. https://well. blogs.nytimes.com/2012/06/06/moderation-as-the-sweet-spot-for-exercise/?_r=0.

———. "Ask Well: Muscle 'Knots'." *The New York Times blog*, July 13, 2015. https://well.blogs.nytimes.com/2015/07/13/experts-divided-on-makeup-and-treatment-of-muscle-knots/?_r=0.

———. "Rethinking the Exercise 'Talk Test'." *The New York Times blog*, September 21, 2011. https://well.blogs.nytimes.com/2011/09/21/rethinking-the-exercise-talk-test/.

Ristevski, Sonja. "Do Foam Rollers Actually Work? A Review of the Evidence." Healthy But Smart. Updated May 3, 2018. https://healthybutsmart.com/foam-rollers/.

Sawicki, George S., Peter Sheppard, and Thomas J. Roberts. "Power Amplification in an Isolated Muscle-Tendon Unit Is Load Dependent." *Journal of Experimental Biology* 218 (2015): 3700–3709. https://doi.org/10.1242/jeb.126235.

Sawicki, Gregory S., Cara L. Lewis, and Daniel P. Ferris. "It Pays to Have a Spring in Your Step." *Exercise and Sport Sciences Reviews* 37, no. 3 (Jul 2009): 130. http://doi.org/10.1097/JES.0b013e31819c2df6.

"Scapulohumeral Rhythm." YouTube, uploaded by Educom Continuing Education, September 11, 2013. https://www.youtube.com/watch?v=H4nfQEeJmFo.

Schaaff, Sarah Vander. "The Strange Pain that Can Overcome Kids, Especially High-Achieving Teenage Girls." *The Washington Post*, August 6, 2017. https://www.washingtonpost.com/national/health-science/the-strange-pain-that-can-overcome-kids-especially-high-achieving-teenage-girls/2017/08/04/2dce9650-659c-11e7-8eb5-cbccc2e7bfbf_story.html?noredirect=on&utm_term=.7c9aaa42bfed.

Schoenfeld, Brad J., and Bret Contreras. "Is Postexercise Muscle Soreness a Valid Indicator of Muscular Adaptations?" *Strength and Conditioning Journal* 35, no. 5 (Oct 2013): 16–21, https://doi.org/10.1519/SSC.0b013e3182a61820.

Schuenke, M. D. et al. "A Description of the Lumbar Interfascial Triangle and Its Relation with the Lateral Raphe: Anatomical Constituents of Load Transfer through the Lateral Margin of the Thoracolumbar Fascia." *Journal of Anatomy* 221, no.6 (Dec 2012): 568–76. http://doi.org/10.1111/j.1469-7580.2012.01517.x.

Scientific American. "Laugh So You Don't Cry: How Laughing Kills the Pain." *The Scicurious Brain* (blog), November 8, 2011. https://blogs.scientificamerican.com/scicurious-brain/laugh-so-you-dont-cry-how-laughing-kills-the-pain/.

Scott, Jonathon P. R., Lars R. McNaughton, and Remco C. J. Polman. "Effects of Sleep Deprivation and Exercise on Cognitive, Motor Performance and Mood." *Physiology & Behavior* 87, no. 2 (Feb 2006): 396–408. https://doi.org/10.1016/j.physbeh.2005.11.009.

Searing, Linda. "Tai Chi, a Chinese Gentle Movement Exercise, May Ease Chronic Disease." *Washington Post*, September 21, 2015. https://www.washingtonpost.com/national/health-science/tai-chi-a-chinese-gentle-movement-exercise-may-ease-chronic-disease/2015/09/21/3b6f43ee-5d66-11e5-b38e-06883aacba64_story.html?utm_term=.8ad50a7877a4.

Shadwick, R. E. "Elastic Energy Storage in Tendons: Mechanical Differences Related to Function and Age." *Journal of Applied Physiology* 68, no. 3 (Mar 1990): 1033–40. https://doi.org/10.1152/jappl.1990.68.3.1033.

Shuchang, He et al. "Emotional and Neurobehavioural Status in Chronic Pain Patients." *Pain Research and Management* 16, no. 1 (2011): 41–43. www.ncbi.nlm.nih.gov/pmc/articles/PMC3052406/.

Shurkin, Joel N. "Trouble Sleeping? Go Camping." *Scientific American*, August 2, 2013. www.scientificamerican.com/article/trouble-sleeping-go-campi/.

Sifferlin, Alexandra. "Why Stretching May Not Help Before Exercise." *Time*, Apr. 8, 2013, healthland.time.com/2013/04/08/why-stretching-may-not-help-before-exercise/.

Smedley, Tim. "What Impact Do Seas, Lakes and Rivers Have on People's Health?" *The Guardian*, March 15, 2013. https://www.theguardian.com/sustainable-business/impact-sea-lakes-rivers-peoples-health.

Smith, M. D., A. Russell, and P. W. Hodges. "Disorders of Breathing and Continence Have a Stronger Association with Back Pain than Obesity and Physical Activity." *Australian Journal of Physiotherapy* 52, no. 1 (2006): 11–16. https://doi.org/10.1016/S0004-9514(06)70057-5.

Smith, Michael T., and Jennifer A. Haythornthwaite. "How Do Sleep Disturbance and Chronic Pain Inter-Relate? Insights from the Longitudinal and Cognitive-Behavioral Clinical Trials Literature." *Sleep Medicine Reviews* 8, no. 2 (Apr 2004): 119–32. https://doi.org/10.1016/S1087-0792(03)00044-3.

Specter, Michael. "The Power of Nothing." *The New Yorker*, December 12, 2011. https://www.newyorker.com/magazine/2011/12/12/the-power-of-nothing.

Sternbergh, Adam. "You Walk Wrong." *New York Magazine*, April 21, 2008. nymag.com/health/features/46213/.

Thatcher, Jon. "Think You Need Back Surgery? Listen to Your Leg Pain." Brattleboro Memorial Hospital. Accessed July 2018. https://www.bmhvt.org/think-you-need-back-surgery-listen-to-your-leg-pain/.

Townsend, George Alfred. "Recreations of Eminent Men." The Chautauquan 15 no. 6 (Apr-Sept 1982): 583. https://books.google.com/books?id=yGQXAQAAIAAJ&pg=PA583&lpg=PA583&dq=#v=onepage&q&f=false

Thomas Jefferson Foundation. "Exercise." Thomas Jefferson Encyclopedia. Accessed March 2017. www.monticello.org/site/research-and-collections/exercise.

Treede, Rolf-Detlef et al. "A Classification of Chronic Pain for ICD-11." Pain 156, no. 6 (Jun 2015): 1003–7. http://doi.org/10.1097/j.pain.0000000000000160.

Tuck Sleep. "Cytokines, Sleep Regulation and Immune Response." Updated February 5, 2018. https://www.tuck.com/cytokines/.

Twin Cities Public Television. "Benjamin Franklin: Inquiring Mind." PBS, 2002. www.pbs.org/benfranklin/l3_inquiring_medical.html.

"UConn Talks—Michael Turvey." YouTube, uploaded by UConn, May 6, 2014. https://www.youtube.com/watch?v=ocZzrIJRGCM.

United States Marine Corps Life. "Marine Corps Looking at Phasing out Sit Ups from PT Tests." Bright Mountain, December 22, 2015. www.usmclife.com/2015/12/marine-corps-looking-phasing-sit-ups-pt-tests/.

University of Pittsburgh Medical Center. "Pitt Research Provides New Insights into How the Mind Influences the Body." August 15, 2016. https://www.upmc.com/media/NewsReleases/2016/Pages/strick-stress-research.aspx.

Van Cauter, Eve, and Laurence Plat. Physiology of Growth Hormone Secretion During Sleep. The Journal of Pediatrics 128, no. 5 (May 1996): S32–S37. https://doi.org/10.1016/S0022-3476(96)70008-2.

Voss, Meagen. "Why High Heels Hurt Even After You Take Them Off." NPR, July 15, 2010. https://www.npr.org/sections/health-shots/2010/07/15/128542551/high-heels-can-make-your-calf-muscles-short.

Voytek, Bradley. "Are There Really as Many Neurons in the Human Brain as Stars in the Milky Way?" Nature. Scitable by Nature Education, May 20, 2013. https://www.nature.com/scitable/blog/brain-metrics/are_there_really_as_many.

WBUR. "Doctor's Orders: For Back Pain, Exercise." June 1, 2017. www.wbur.org/onpoint/2017/06/01/doctors-back-pain-exercise.

WebMD. "The Healing Power of Sleep." Updated October 6, 2016. www.webmd.com/a-to-z-guides/discomfort-15/better-sleep/healing-power-sleep?page=2.

Weingart, Heidi M., and Len Kravitz. "Resistance Training and Bone Mass." The University of New Mexico, 2001. https://www.unm.edu/~lkravitz/Article%20folder/bonemass.html.

Willard, F. H. et al. "The Thoracolumbar Fascia: Anatomy, Function and Clinical Considerations." Journal of Anatomy 221, no.6 (May 2012): 507–36. http://doi.org/10.1111/j.1469-7580.2012.01511.x.

Williams, Lawrence E., and John A. Bargh. "Experiencing Physical Warmth Promotes Interpersonal Warmth." Science 322, no. 5901 (Oct 2008): 606–7. http://doi.org/10.1126/science.1162548.

Wolff, Phillip, and Jason Shepard. "Causation, Touch, and the Perception of Force." Psychology of Learning and Motivation 58 (Dec 2013). https://doi.org/10.1016/B978-0-12-407237-4.00005-0.

Wolford, Monica L., Kathleen Palso, and Anita Bercovitz. "Hospitalization for Total Hip Replacement Among Inpatients Aged 45 and Over: United States, 2000–2010." NCHS Date Brief No. 186. February 2015. https://www.cdc.gov/nchs/products/databriefs/db186.htm.

Woodham, Mark et al. "Long-Term Lumbar Multifidus Muscle Atrophy Changes Documented with Magnetic Resonance Imaging: A Case Series." Journal of Radiology Case Reports 8, no. 5 (May 2014): 27–34. http://doi.org/10.3941/jrcr.v8i5.1401.

World Heritage Encyclopedia. s.v. "Unconscious Proprioception." Project Gutenberg Self-Publishing Press, 2018. www.self.gutenberg.org/articles/Unconscious_proprioception.

Yeager, Selene. "The Secret to Being Fit for Life: Muscle Memory." Women's Health Magazine. Hearst Communications, November 9, 2010. https://www.womenshealthmag.com/style/a19900844/fit-for-life/.

Zielinski, Mark R. "Sleep and Inflammation—Intimate Partners in Health and Functioning." Thrive Global, May 16, 2017. https://medium.com/thrive-global/the-fascinating-link-between-inflammation-and-sleep-9d57c2eca013.